THE WHAT'S HAPPENING TO MY BODY?
BOOK FOR BOYS

OTHER BOOKS BY LYNDA MADARAS

My Body, My Self for Boys
with Area Madaras

My Body, My Self for Girls
with Area Madaras

My Feelings, My Self: A Growing-Up Guide for Girls
with Area Madaras

The What's Happening to My Body? Book for Girls
with Area Madaras

*Lynda Madaras Talks to Teens About AIDS: An Essential Guide
for Parents, Teachers, and Young People*

Womancare: A Gynecological Guide to Your Body
with Jane Patterson, M.D.

Woman Doctor: The Education of Jane Patterson, M.D.,
with Jane Patterson, M.D.

Great Expectations with Leigh Adams

The Alphabet Connection with Pam Palewicz-Rousseau

Child's Play

THE WHAT'S HAPPENING TO MY BODY? BOOK FOR BOYS

THIRD EDITION
A Growing-Up Guide for Parents and Sons

LYNDA MADARAS
WITH AREA MADARAS

*Drawings by Simon Sullivan
and Jackie Aher*

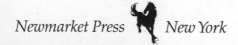

Newmarket Press • New York

Library of Congress Cataloging-in-Publication Data

Madaras, Lynda.
    The "what's happening to my body?" book for boys : a growing-up
    guide for parents and sons / Lynda Madaras, with Area Madaras ;
    drawings by Simon Sullivan and Jackie Aher.—3rd ed.
        p. cm.
    Includes bibliographical references and index.
    Summary: Discusses the changes that take place in a boy's body
during puberty, including information on the body's changing size and
shape, the growth spurt, reproductive organs, pubic hair, beards, pimples,
voice changes, wet dreams, and puberty in girls.
    ISBN 1-55704-443-0 (pbk.)—ISBN 1-55704-447-3 (hc.)
    1. Teenage boys—Growth—Juvenile literature. 2. Teenage boyls—
Physiology—Juvenile literature. 3. Puberty—Juvenile literature.
    4. Sex instruction for boys—Juvenile literature. [1. Teenage boys.
    2. Puberty. 3. Sex instruction for boys.] I. Madaras, Area.
    II. Aher, Jackie, ill. III. Sullivan, Simon, ill. IV. Title.

        RJ143 .M33 2000
        613.9'53—dc21   00-031873

QUANTITY PURCHASES
Companies, professional groups, clubs, and other organizations
may qualify for special terms when ordering quantities of this title.
For information contact Newmarket Press, Special Sales Department,
18 East 48th Street, New York, NY 10017; phone 212-832-3575;
fax 212-832-3629; or e-mail sales@newmarketpress.com.

Website: www.newmarketpress.com

Manufactured in the United States of America
THIRD EDITION
9   8   7   6   5   4   3   2   1

CONTENTS

LIST OF ILLUSTRATIONS

FOREWORD BY
MARTIN ANDERSON, M.D., M.P.H.

Unfortunately, teenagers don't come equipped with owners' manuals like new cars do. Both are high performance, occasionally high maintenance, and can be difficult to start, steer, and stop. One major roadblock in parent-teen communication is that each side doesn't know what to expect from the other. Parents usually teach their children based on how they themselves were taught. This works well for throwing a ball, fishing, changing the oil in a car, cooking, etc., but fails in the area of sexuality and pubertal development. Parents often weren't taught these subjects by their own parents and therefore they have no model to draw from when teaching their children.

Lynda Madaras's book functions equally well as an owner's manual for teens and as a teaching guide for their parents. I strongly agree with the author when she suggests that this book should be read by parents and teens/pre-teens together. This informative volume prepares both teens and their parents for the changes that are coming, and the book is a great resource for teens later on when they have questions about their bodies.

I have had the pleasure of leading several father/son sessions on puberty/growth-development for fifth-grade boys and their dads. The substance of the presentations and what transpires during the sessions are far less important than discussions that occur on the way home and later. Parents and their teens often need something to initiate these discussions. Lynda Madaras's book is an excellent starting place for these discussions.

For teens reading this, remember that parents are often just as uncomfortable, if not more so than you are. Believe it or not, they went through puberty just as you are now. Ask them about their experiences. You might just learn something and, if not, think of the embarrassing information you will find out about your parents. Now you can get even with them for showing your naked baby pictures to your first date.

In summary Lynda Madaras's book is an invaluable resource for teens and their parents. Both teens and their parents can benefit a great deal from reading this book. It is one of the classic books I keep on hand to lend parents or teens when they ask for resources to help understand adolescence.

Martin Anderson, M.D., M.P.H.
Director of Adolescent Medicine
UCLA Department of Pediatrics
Los Angeles, California

INTRODUCTION FOR PARENTS: WHY I WROTE THIS BOOK

Toward the end of the school year, I give each of the boys and girls in my sex-education classes a raw egg and a homework assignment that goes something like this:

We're going to play a game. For one week, this egg is your baby. Fortunately for you, you don't have to feed it or change its diapers or get a job in order to earn enough money to buy clothes for it and put a roof over its head. But other than this, you have to take care of the egg as if it really were a baby and you were responsible for it. This means that you can't leave it alone unless you arrange for someone else to watch it while you're gone.

I'm giving you a break, though. I'm going to say that your babies are old enough to sleep through the night. This means that your baby won't wake up at two or three in the morning, howling to be fed—an unfortunate habit that most real babies have during the first months of their lives.

As I say, your babies are old enough to sleep through the night, so all you have to do at bedtime is give baby a kiss and tuck him or her (you decide which it is) into the refrigerator. You don't have to worry about baby again until the next morning. But in the morning, you have to remember to take your baby out of the fridge and bring it to school.

When you forget to bring your lunch money or gym clothes or math book to school, nothing too terrible happens. But if you forget to bring your baby to school even once, it's dead and you're out of the game. Not only that, but if any member of the Child Welfare League finds a neglected baby—that is, a baby left unattended—that baby will be confiscated.

I am president of the Child Welfare League, and all the staff and teachers are members. So is every student in the school, which means that you, too, are a member of the League. You are sworn to protect the welfare of all egg babies, and as your president, I expect every member of the League to be extremely vigilant about confiscating unattended and neglected babies.

At the end of the week, I will take all surviving babies and their parents out to lunch.

Good luck!

P.S. The parents of confiscated babies will not be taken to lunch.

The egg babies in my classes do not fare well. Most die of multiple fractures soon after birth. Some rot. Others simply disappear in the eternity of time that is a child's week. Still others are confiscated by the alarmingly zealous junior members of the Child Welfare League.

One year there was even a baby who committed suicide—at least that's how the baby's "father" attempted to explain the demise of his egg. It seems this baby had, "all by itself," totally of its own accord, rolled off his desk in the middle of French class. The father tried to argue that the parent of a suicidal baby deserved to be taken out to lunch. Being a hard-hearted lot, the class refused to acknowledge his point.

I must admit that I get a real kick out of watching what goes on at school in the week during this homework assignment. There are always a couple of boys who try to get one of the girls to care for their babies because "taking care of babies is women's work." It warms the cockles of my heart to see this tactic fall flat on its face. But there are also the boys who take their parenting very seriously. I'll see them out on the patio at lunch, four or five boys eating together, with their egg babies resting on a strip of soft velvet in the center of the table. They'll be chatting away about the various bumps and cracks their babies have just narrowly escaped, sounding for all the world like the congregations of young mothers who gather over baby strollers in the park to compare notes and trade tales of barely averted childhood disasters.

Within a day or so after I have given the assignment, the egg babies have taken on definite personalities. Carefully crayoned features appear on their formerly blank faces, and the "parents" have all named their babies. Ingenious cribs and cradles and carriages have been fashioned. Once, a boy brought his egg to school in a plastic, oval panty-hose container—a "self-contained life-support capsule," the proud father explained.

It always surprises me that it is not just the younger kids but also the older teens—and the boys as well as the girls—who get involved in the game and set about designing these cribs and cradles and such for their babies. The sight of a hulking fifteen-year-old with the build of a football player trotting across the campus with his egg baby tenderly tucked in a carefully constructed milk carton cradle never fails to amaze me.

This homework assignment comes at the end of a section of the curriculum in which the kids, at least the ones in my older classes, tackle such thorny issues as:

- How old should you be before you have sex?
- How do you know if you're ready for sex?
- Should you wait until you're married?
- How to say no to sex
- Birth control
- The fact that birth control isn't 100 percent effective
- Abortion

- Parenthood
- Sexuality and the responsibility for the lives and feelings of others

The thinking behind the egg baby assignment is, of course, to give kids some idea of the realities of and the responsibilities involved in parenthood. I suppose that, at the heart of it, this assignment is really nothing more than an old-fashioned moral object lesson, something along the lines of the stories my grandmother would tell in which children, although warned not to, would skate on thin-ice ponds and drown. Although I heard these tales often, I did venture out on a few thin-ice ponds in my time, and, all in all, the warnings did not have a profound effect on me. So I am not naive enough to think that giving kids raw eggs to take care of for a week is going to make them stop in the middle of the throes of teenage passion and think about forgoing sex altogether or at least using birth control. Still, I figure it can't hurt. We do, after all, have a virtual epidemic of teenage pregnancies in this country. Over a million babies are born to teenage mothers each year—that's one in every nine girls aged fifteen to nineteen and one in five who are sexually active. Given these facts, anything—even a long shot like the egg baby assignment—seems worth a try.

Even if this assignment never prevents a single teenage pregnancy, the kids have fun and I like to think they learn something from it. But more important, perhaps, is that each year I learn, or relearn, something about the confusing contradictions young boys must deal with as they move into manhood.

The boys who are out on the patio clucking over their babies, the football players who have spent hours lovingly fashioning their cribs and cradles, are the very same boys who come up to me before class, giggling and pushing at me dog-eared copies of whatever racy, adolescent paperback novel has been making the rounds of late. "Read this, read this," they insist, the books open to pages on which "the good parts" have been underlined in red.

For many years, it was Nick Carter novels. Possibly you aren't familiar with Nick. I myself have never read much more than "the good parts" of any Nick Carter novel. Apparently, though, Nick is some sort of detective or international spy or CIA operative. Nick and his fellow heroes of this particular literary genre are quite a bunch of guys. They have all sorts of thrilling adventures and narrow escapes. They are, each and every one, precision marksmen. They generally drive very fast, very expensive, very red sports cars. They are well versed in obscure martial arts, which they regularly apply to various thugs and scoundrels of a vaguely Mafioso, Communist ilk. And, of course, truth, justice, the American way, and our heroes always triumph in the end. But all the intrigue and rather convoluted plots are just so much window dressing, merely something to hang "the good parts" on—for what the Nick Carter novels and the others of the genre are really about is *sex*.

Curiously enough, Nick and his literary counterparts, at least in my spotty readings, rarely seem to make the first sexual moves. Instead, it's the women who "come on" to them (a rather effective device for sidestepping the old fear-of-rejection problem).

There is nothing in the least bit shy or retiring about the ladies Nick encounters. They are a most lascivious lot. The women in these novels are forever ripping open their blouses and begging our hero to have his way with them. The hero, being a gentleman, obliges. There is a curiously Victorian coyness to the lurid detailing of these sexual exploits. It's always the hero's "manhood," his "organ," his "hardness," or his throbbing pulsating "member" that so delights the ladies and their "wet openness"—never anything so clinical, explicit, or mundane as a "penis" or a "vagina."

These sexual gymnastics often continue for several pages. As I said, Nick and his cohorts are quite a bunch of guys. Often the episodes wind to a close with the ladies expressing gratitude for the wonderful satisfaction our hero has provided and declaring their undying love for him, although as far as I've been able to determine the women and the hero rarely, if ever, meet up again.

I am not normally one to rain on anybody's parade, but when the boys in my classes ask me to read the underlined sections of books like these, I figure that they're asking for some sort of reaction, that they want to know what I think. So I tell them. I do my best to avoid being sarcastic—that clearly isn't the tack called for here. I explain that neither my sex life nor the sex life of anyone else I know on the planet proceeds along the lines described in these books. We discuss what's unreal about the sexual encounters in Nick's life and why the author chose to portray them in this light. We talk about the real-life fears and uncertainties most people have in regard to sex, about sexuality, and the emotional feelings involved in being sexual with another person. From an educational point of view, we get a lot of mileage out of old Nick.

The issue I'm trying to get at here is that this culture poses some rather tricky problems for young boys trying to find their way into manhood. On the one hand, they have a tender, caring side—the side I see so clearly when they're essentially "playing dolls" with egg babies.

On the other hand, they are confronted with all these thrilling and titillating images of a conquering, tough-guy male sexuality, which doesn't seem to allow much room for anybody's being at all tender or caring. It must be rather difficult to reconcile making a cradle for your egg baby with the sagas of Nick Carter. It must be very hard for a boy to sort all this out, and this undoubtedly accounts for a large portion of the adolescent male angst. Of course, what I'm talking about here isn't any great revelation. We all know that during childhood boys generally are allowed some room, given some social permission, to demonstrate or act out their tender side. But at adolescence they move into the strange world of male adulthood in which, if Nick is to be believed, "real men" are not noted for their tenderness, "real men" don't cry or ever feel uncertain about who they are or what they're supposed to do, "real men" always know the right sexual moves to make, "real men" are always knowledgeable and supremely confident about sex and life in general. Whew!

To top it all off, just as they're moving from childhood into this confusing world of manhood, all these strange changes start happening to their bodies. And chances are that nobody around them seems willing to explain these changes in any but the most cursory way, if at all. In fact, the message that boys are getting is that somehow they're supposed to *know* about these things, for one of the main tenets of the male mystique is that guys, or at least "real men," automatically know everything about anything that has to do with sex.

Most of the girls in my classes have been the recipients of at least one rather nervous and embarrassed "talk" from their parents (as a rule, their mothers) about menstruation, the hallmark of female puberty. But there are very few boys in my classes whose parents (either the mother or the father) have talked with them about ejaculation, the hallmark of male puberty, or about spontaneous erections, masturbation, wet dreams, or any of the other physical realities of male puberty. As a culture, we seem to have decided that it's important to talk to our daughters about puberty but not so important to talk to our sons.

Of course, it's a lot easier to ignore our sons' "coming of age" than it is to ignore our daughters'. A daughter's first menstruation requires at least some minimal parental response. Someone's got to buy her a box of sanitary napkins or tampons and tell her how they're used and not to flush them down the toilet. When a boy ejaculates for the first time, we don't have to rush out to the store for anything or worry about him clogging up the plumbing.

There's also the fact that once our daughters begin to menstruate regularly, they become capable of getting pregnant. This fact alone seems to convince many parents that there ought to be at least some minimal discussion of a daughter's sexual changes. (And yet, girls don't get pregnant by themselves. As my mother used to say, "It takes two to tango," although she was never talking about dancing when she said this.)

Or maybe it's just the old male mystique, the belief that boys automatically know everything they need to know about sex. Few parents would actually argue that boys will magically understand what's happening to their bodies without someone telling them. But many parents have the attitude that puberty isn't really a "big deal" for boys. There's a popular idea in our culture that it's only girls who are embarrassed, anxious, and worried about the physical changes of puberty.

You couldn't prove it by me. I get hundreds and hundreds of letters from boys who've read my books, the envelopes covered with underscored pleas—"Help!", "URGENT!,""Open At Once!,""Please! Please! Write Back Right Away!!!" Inside there'll be five-page letters with intricate diagrams and lengthy explanations of some lump or bump or imagined physical abnormality that has the poor kid worried sick. (The volume of mail from boys is nearly equal to that from girls.)

In my classes, we play a game called *Everything You Ever Wanted to Know About Sex and Puberty But Were Too Embarrassed to Ask*, which involves a locked question box to which kids can anonymously submit questions. At the end of each class, I open the box, read out loud the questions that have accumulated that week, and answer them as best I can. The questions come printed in block letters (to disguise the handwriting), and the paper on which they're written has inevitably been folded about ten times into a tiny little packet. After all, this is embarrassing stuff.

Judging from the questions that come up, boys are just as curious as girls about what's happening to their bodies. For every question about menstrual periods or developing breasts, there's one about wet dreams, ejaculations, or hair growth, things like, "How much of that white stuff comes out when a guy comes?" and "When will I grow a beard and start to look like my dad?"Here's just one example:

> I am growing a mustash. Not a big mustash, but tiny hares. How can a boy by the age of eleven? He didn't have puberty yet.

The spelling and syntax are unusual, but the spirit behind the question isn't. This boy was worried about the fact that he was developing some fine hairs on his upper lip but he'd never "had puberty," by which he meant that he hadn't ever ejaculated. Generally, facial hair doesn't appear until the sex organs are fairly well developed, the boy's begun making sperm in his testicles, and he's already begun to ejaculate. But boys develop in different ways, and although it's *unusual* to develop a mustache before these other changes have begun to occur, it's certainly not *abnormal.* This boy, like most young boys, was simply looking for reassurance that what was happening to him was completely normal. It seems little enough to ask.

Yet far too many parents leave their sons adrift at this important time in their lives. One factor in our failure to talk to our sons about the physical changes of puberty is undoubtedly simple ignorance. Most fathers didn't get much information from their own fathers. They don't exactly have a storehouse of knowledge to pass on to their sons. Although they have a general idea of what happens during puberty— having gone through it themselves— it's a rare father who can explain to his son exactly why he might have wet dreams or tell him the average age at which a boy first ejaculates. Mothers are at even more of a loss in this respect. They might feel confident enough to make a stab at telling a daughter about menstruation; after all, they've been menstruating themselves for most of their lives. But when it comes to spontaneous erections, wet dreams, and such, they're generally completely at sea.

Another factor in most parents' failure to tell their sons about the body changes of puberty is embarrassment. Sexuality is a difficult, even nigh on to impossible topic for many parents. Even those of us who feel fairly easy about discussing sex may find that there are certain areas of sexuality that we're not entirely comfortable talking over with our children. Take masturbation, for example. It's pretty difficult to discuss puberty with a boy without talking about masturbation. Over 90 percent of boys masturbate during puberty. Yet masturbation is a delicate subject, and most of us are bound to feel a little embarrassed discussing it. For one thing, how in the world do you even broach the subject in the first place? What do you say? "Hi, son, been masturbating lately?"

As you may have guessed, I'm coming around to the why-I-wrote-the-book part of this introduction. The purpose of the book is, of course, to provide the basic information that young boys want and need about what's happening to their bodies as they go through puberty, information that we as parents all too often don't have available to give them. Beyond providing the basic facts, I hope that the book will help parents and sons get past the "embarrassment barrier." Ideally, I imagine parents (both the father and the mother) sitting down and reading the book with their sons. Somehow, having the facts printed on a page makes it less embarrassing—someone else is saying it, not you; you're just reading the information.

Of course, it's not necessary for both parents to read the book with their son. Either one parent or the other may choose to do so, or it may work better in your particular situation for you to simply give the book to your son to read on his own. You may not even have to give it to him. Parents often tell me that they've bought my books intending to read them with their child. But, before they'd gotten around to it, the child has found the book lying around the house and is already halfway through it.

Regardless of whether you read it separately or together, I hope you'll find a way to talk with your son about the changes that are—or soon will be—taking place in his body. Kids often have minute and detailed concerns about these changes. They need lots of reassurance that what's happening to them is perfectly normal. It's been my experience that kids are enormously grateful for such reassurance. I actually have had classes where kids burst into spontaneous applause when I walked into the room. I also have file drawers full of touching letters from readers thanking me for having allayed some fear or doubt of theirs.

Not only are kids grateful when their needs for reassurance are met in this way, but they also develop a profound respect for and trust in the source of that reassurance. Parents need to realize what a powerful bond they can forge with their sons if they will "be there" for them during puberty—not to mention how well the ensuing trust and respect will serve all concerned in later years when your son is making decisions about sex. If you're there for your kid when he's wondering, he's more likely to come to you for advice when he's deciding.

Having said all this, I should also warn you that, even after your son has read the book, talking about puberty changes with your son may not be the easiest thing to do. If you come at it head-on by asking a direct question—"What did you think of the book?" or "Is there anything in the book you'd like to talk about?"—it's possible that you'll get a wonderfully detailed critical appraisal of the book, or a series of open, frank questions. What's more likely, though, is that you'll get something along the lines of, "It was okay," or "Naw, there's nothin' I want to know," or "I donwanna talk about that stuff."

In my experience, it's better to take a slightly different approach. Start things off by saying something along these lines:

"Gee, when I was about your age, I _____."

(Fill in the blank:"noticed my first hairs," "had my first wet dream," "ejaculated for the first time," or whatever.)

"I felt really_____("nervous," "excited," "proud," "embarrassed," "afraid," or whatever).

"In fact, what happened to me was that I _____ _____." (Again, fill in the blank with a story about something from your own adolescence, the more embarrassing or stupid the story, the better.)

By using this approach, you make it easier for your kid to open up. By virtue of whatever embarrassing, dumb story you've told about yourself, you've let your kid know that it's okay to be uncertain and less than all-knowingly perfect about the whole business. At least the kids in my class always seem to open up when I tell them about things like:

The time I bet my best friend, Georgia, my entire allowance that the way people had babies was: the man kissed the woman; a seed from his belly came up his throat, went into her mouth and down her throat, landing in her belly; and nine months later, a baby came out of her belly button. I lost my entire allowance to Georgia.

Or the time my brother ran for class president and had to give a speech in the auditorium in front of everyone in the whole school, and got a spontaneous erection and didn't know if everyone was laughing at the jokes in his speech or the fact that he had a hard-on.

You get the idea.

Here's another pearl of wisdom: avoid having one all-purpose talk. It won't fill the bill, no matter how hard you try. It's also better to approach things casually, bringing up the topic from time to time when it seems natural to do so. When I was beginning puberty, my mother sat me down one day to have the Talk. I'm sure she must have explained things in a fairly comprehensible way. All I recall, though, was my mother being horribly nervous and embarrassed and saying a lot of stuff about blood and babies. Then she said something about how when it happened to me, I could come and get some napkins out of the bottom drawer of her bedroom dresser. I remember wondering why in the world she'd be keeping napkins in the bottom drawer of her dresser instead of the top drawer of the kitchen cabinet, which was where napkins were normally kept in our house. But my mother was acting so weird that it just didn't seem like the kind of question to ask at the time. In my experience, a more casual, spur-of-the-moment approach to talking to your child about puberty works better.

Yet another piece of advice: if talking about puberty and sexuality is difficult or embarrassing for you, say so. There's nothing wrong with telling your child, "This is really embarrassing for me," or "My parents never talked to me about this stuff, so I feel kind of weird trying to talk to you," or whatever. Your child is going to pick up on your embarrassment anyway from your tone of voice, your body language, or any one of the other ways we have of communicating what we're really feeling. By trying to pretend you're not uncomfortable, you'll only succeed in confusing your child. Once you've admitted your feelings, you've cleared the air. Your child may adopt a maddeningly smug attitude or be patronizingly sympathetic about your embarrassment, but in the end this is preferable to having him think that there is something weird about the topic itself, that it's not quite right to talk about it.

The book you have here was designed for boys in the nine- to fifteen-year-old group, although it may be appropriate for younger or older boys as well. I hope the book is one that you'll reread with your son time and again as he's growing older, or that you'll keep around the house so that he can go back to it. What a child of eight or nine takes away from this book will be different from what a boy of thirteen or fourteen does. For example, Chapters 6 and 7 deal with spontaneous erections, ejaculations, wet dreams, and masturbation. In my experience, boys of nine or ten are quite curious about these topics, even though they may not have their first wet dreams and ejaculations until they are thirteen, fourteen, or older. In fact, younger boys are often more open and easy about discussing these topics than they will be a few years later, when they are experiencing them. At nine or ten, a boy may read these chapters and take away a certain understanding. But, at age thirteen or fourteen, when these things are much more real and immediate, the information will be meaningful in different ways. It's important that a boy be prepared for the pubertal changes described in this book before they happen, but it's also important that he be able to go back and reread the information after these changes have started to take place in his own body.

As a parent, you may find that you have some concerns about some of the material covered in this book. Some of the topics are very controversial. When controversial questions come up in class, I try to present the various points of view and explain why people have them. I think I do a pretty good job of being objective, but sometimes my own point of view comes through. For instance, when discussing masturbation, I explain that some people feel it is wrong or sinful and not at all a good thing to do, and I talk about why they feel that way. But the truth of the matter is that I feel very strongly that masturbation is a perfectly fine, perfectly normal thing to do, and I'm sure that this comes through in what I've written. You may find that your opinions on masturbation or some of the other topics covered in this book are different from mine, but this doesn't mean you have to throw the baby out with the bathwater. Instead, you can use these differences as an opportunity to explain and elucidate your own attitudes and values to your child.

Regardless of how you decide to deal with the topics of puberty and sexuality or how you decide to use this book, I hope that it will help you and your child to gain a greater understanding of the process of puberty and that it will bring the two of you closer together.

ADDENDUM TO THE THIRD EDITION

This third edition differs from the previous edition in a number of ways. Some of the chapters have been reorganized and a good deal of new material has been added. For example, there is a new chapter, "An Owner's Guide to the Male Sex Organs: What's Normal? What's Not?" The chapter includes a more detailed discussion of penis size, an issue that—judging from the letters I get—seems to obsess the male psyche. Indeed, I get more letters from male readers dealing with questions and concerns about penis size than about all other topics combined. I hope the new material on penis size in Chapter 3 will set a few minds to rest.

Chapter 3 also includes new material on the anatomy and function of the foreskin and the care of the uncircumcised penis. In the past, nearly all male babies born in this country were circumcised. Over the years, things have changed. Today only about 60 percent of babies are circumcised in the United States. More boys than ever are reaching puberty with their foreskins still intact. Basic, everyday knowledge about the foreskin and its care used to be handed down from father to son. With so many men being circumcised in this country, much of the knowledge was lost. Thus, boys with their foreskins intact often have unanswered questions about their bodies. In addition, the foreskin has pretty much disappeared from medical textbooks. Doctors in the United States often know little about the foreskin except how to remove it. The result is that all too often minor foreskin irritations are treated rather drastically—by surgical removal. I hope the new information in Chapter 3 will not only help answer boys' questions, but will also help them hang on to their foreskins should problems arise.

The chapter on the growth during puberty has been expanded. In response to questions from readers and boys in my workshops and classes, I have included information on weight training during puberty and steroid abuse. Studies showing that American kids are turning into couch potatoes and that adolescent boys get only about half the calcium they need prompted me to add a section called "Eating Right and Exercising" to this chapter.

Throughout the book, material has been updated and expanded to respond to new research and developments. For example, there is new material on the causes and treatment of acne. In addition, input from the boys and men in my classes and workshops and from readers' letters has led me to expand the material on certain topics. For instance, there is more discussion of ejaculation, in particular the first ejaculations a boy experiences during puberty. (I've also endeavored to make the information on shaving less "girly" and more pertinent to male shaving needs.)

Throughout the book I have made a systematic effort to simplify sentence structure and vocabulary. This makes the book easier for younger boys to read. At the same time I have been careful not to skip details or to sacrifice accuracy.

In the second edition of this book there are two chapters dealing with sexual intercourse, pregnancy, birth control, and sexually transmitted diseases. I have removed these two chapters and presented only a minimum of information about these topics in this edition. However, in the Resource Section of this edition I do point boys to additional information on these topics. Quite frankly, I did think that the second edition was a bit on the long side. Now, with both younger readers and new material on puberty education issues, the inclusion of two full chapters on sex education issues would have made this new edition quite a long tome.

This shortening of the sex education material included in this book is consistent with my overall understanding of the strong need for early puberty education. To quote from my second edition, and I hope without seeming to be pompous, "Kids who aren't given reassuring puberty education when they need it do not respond as well to their parents' or schools' efforts to impart moral codes or even just safe, sane guidelines for sexual conduct." Sex education may help allay our own fears about pregnancies and STDs, but first we must reassure our kids about the changes happening to their bodies during puberty.

I hope this book will help you reassure your son and help the two of you develop an even closer and more loving relationship.

CHAPTER 1

Puberty

It was great. I remember thinking, "I'm not just a kid anymore!" I loved it!

John, age 26

It was weird. I was tired all the time and sleeping a whole lot. I wasn't really sure what was happening to me.

Bill, age 19

People make it sound like it's this big dramatic thing that all of a sudden happens one day. It's not like that. It's not like some guy pops up and says, "Hey, kid, this is it. Now it's going to happen to you."

Jackson, age 33

It seemed like I woke up one day and everything had changed. I was a different person in a different body.

Sam, age 35

These men are all talking about the same thing—*puberty.** Puberty is the time in your life when your body is changing from a child's body into an adult's body.

*There are a number of words in this book that we think you may not have heard before. When we first use these words, you'll find a

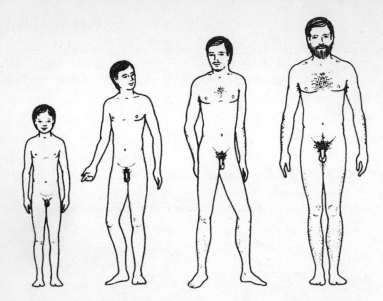

Figure 1. Male Puberty Changes. As boys go through puberty, they get taller, their shoulders get wider, their bodies more muscular, their sex organs develop, and they begin to grow pubic hair, as well as hair on their underarms, faces, chests, arms, and legs.

As you can see from Figure 1, a boy's body changes quite a bit as he goes through puberty. His *penis* and his *scrotum*, the sac of skin just behind his penis, grow and

pronunciation key like this at the bottom of the page. We always use capital letters to indicate which part of the word to emphasize when you say it out loud. And we use "uh" in the pronunciation guide to indicate the vowel sound that rhymes with the "uh" in "huh." See, for example, "vulva," "testicles," and "urethra." Remember that you don't pronounce the "h" in "uh." We also use "ih" to indicate the vowel sound that rhymes with the "e" in "edit."

puberty (PEW-bur-tee) You say puberty with the most emphasis on the first part of the word, PEW.
penis (PEE-niss)
scrotum (SKROW-tum)

develop. Hair grows in places where it never grew before—around his penis, under his arms, and on his face.

A boy also gets taller. Of course, we grow taller all through childhood. But, during puberty, a boy grows taller at a faster rate than he ever will again. During this growth spurt, he may gain four or more inches in one year. The shape of his body changes, too. His shoulders become broader, and his hips then look narrower in comparison. His muscles develop and his body strength increases. His whole body begins to look more "manly."

These are just some of the outward changes in a boy's body during puberty. While these changes are happening on the outside of the body, other changes are already happening on the inside. For some boys, puberty seems to take forever. For others, these changes happen so fast they seem to take place overnight. They don't really happen that quickly, though. Puberty happens slowly and gradually, over a period of many months and years. The first changes may start when a boy is quite young, or may not begin until his teen years. No matter when puberty starts for you, I bet you'll have lots of questions about what's happening to your body. I hope this book will answer those questions.

I teach classes on puberty for kids and for parents. My daughter, Area, and I also do workshops on puberty. The men and boys in our workshops and the boys in my classes always have lots of questions. They also have lots to say about puberty. Their quotes appear throughout these pages.* So, in a sense, they helped write this book.

I first began teaching puberty and sexuality classes back in the days when dinosaurs still roamed the earth

---

* To protect their privacy, we changed the names of the boys and men who were kind enough to let us quote them.

(well, nearly that long ago, anyhow). Back then, sex education wasn't taught in very many schools. I had to invent my lesson plans from scratch. I decided to start off my very first class by explaining how babies are made. This seemed like a good place to begin. After all, during puberty, your body is getting ready for a time in your life when you may decide to reproduce—that is to make a baby.

I didn't think I'd have any problems teaching that first class. "Nothing to it," I told myself. "I'll just go in there and start by talking to the kids about how babies are made. No problem."

Boy, was I wrong! I'd hardly opened my mouth before the class went crazy. Kids were giggling, nudging each other, and getting red in the face. One boy even fell off his chair. The class was acting weird because to talk about how babies are made, I had to talk about sex. Sex, as you may have noticed, is a *very big deal*. People often act embarrassed, giggly, or strange when the topic of sex comes up.

SEX

The word *sex* itself is confusing. Even though it's a small word, *sex* has a lot of meanings. In its most basic meaning, *sex* simply refers to the different bodies males and females have. There are lots of differences between male and female bodies. The most obvious is that males have a penis and a scrotum, and females have a *vulva* and a *vagina*. These body parts, or organs, are called sex organs. People have either male or female sex organs and belong to either the male or female sex.

vulva (VUL-vuh)
vagina (vah-JEYE-nuh)

The word *sex* is also used in other ways. We may say that two people are "having sex." This usually means they are having *sexual intercourse*. As we'll explain later in this chapter, sexual intercourse involves the joining together of two people's sex organs. Intercourse between a male and a female is also how babies are made.

We may say that two people are "being sexual with each other." This means they are having sexual intercourse or are holding, touching, or caressing each other's sex organs. We may say that we are "feeling sexual." This means that we are having feelings or thoughts about our sex organs or about being sexual with another person.

Our sex organs are private parts of our bodies. We usually keep them covered. We don't talk about them in public very often. Having sexual feelings and being sexual with someone aren't usually classroom topics either.

If I had half a brain in my head, I would have thought about all this before my first class. I would have realized that coming into a classroom and talking about sex, penises, and vaginas was going to cause a *big* commotion.

After that first class, I caught on real quick. I decided that, if we were going to get all silly and giggly, we might as well get *really* silly and giggly. Now I start my classes and workshops by passing out copies of the drawings in Figure 2. I also give everyone red and blue colored pencils.

Figure 2 shows the sex organs on the outside of the body in a grown man and a grown woman. These sex organs are also called the *genital*, or *reproductive*, organs.

sexual intercourse (SEK-shoo-uhl IN-ter-kors)
genital (JEN-uh-tuhl)
reproductive (REE-pruh-DUKT-iv)

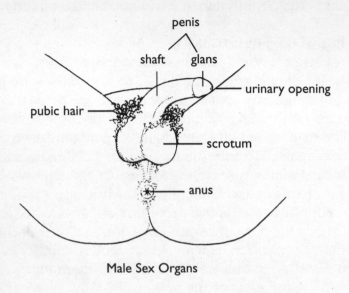

Male Sex Organs

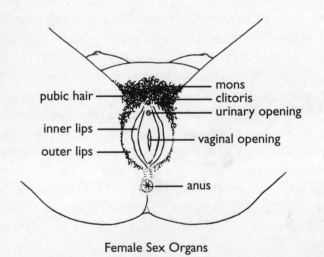

Female Sex Organs

Figure 2. The Sex Organs

We have sex organs on both the inside and outside of our bodies. They change as we go through puberty.

THE MALE SEX ORGANS

Once everyone has copies and colored pencils, I hold up the picture of the male sex organs. I tell the class that the sex organs on the outside of a man's body are the *penis* and the *scrotum*. The kids in my class still giggle like mad or fall off their chairs in embarrassment, but I don't pay much attention. Using my best Kindergarten Lady voice, I say, "The penis itself has two parts: the *shaft* and the *glans*. Find the shaft of the penis and color it with blue and red stripes." Now everybody gets very intent on the coloring. Some are still giggling, but they do start coloring. Why don't you color the shaft in, too? (Unless, of course, this book belongs to someone else or to a library. One of the people we most admire is a librarian named Lou Ann Sobieski. We would be in very hot water if Lou Ann thought we were telling people to color library books. If this book isn't yours, make a copy of the page to color.)

Next I ask the class to find the small slit at the tip of the penis and circle it in red. This is the *urinary* opening. It is the opening through which *urine* (pee) leaves the body. There's usually less giggling by now. The urinary opening is small. The class has to pay more attention to the coloring.

Then we color in the glans itself. I usually suggest blue, but color it any way you want.

glans (GLANZ)
urinary (YOUR-in-air-ee)
urine (YOUR-in)

"Red and blue polka dots for the scrotum," I tell my class next. The scrotum is a loose bag of skin that lies beneath the penis. *Scrotal sac* is another name for the scrotum. Inside the scrotum are two egg-shaped organs called *testes*, or *testicles*. (You can't see the testicles in Figure 2. I mention them because we will be talking about them in just a few pages.)

Then, I explain that the curly hairs on the sex organs are *pubic* hairs. I have the class color them as well.

Finally, we come to the *anus*. This is the opening through which *feces* (*bowel* movements) leave our bodies. The anus isn't a reproductive organ. But it's nearby, so you might as well color it, too.

By the time the class has colored in the different parts, I've said the word *penis* out loud about twenty-eight times. Everyone is used to my saying this and other words that aren't usually said out loud in classrooms. My students no longer have to go crazy each time I use these words. Besides, the pictures look funny. Everyone is laughing. Laughter makes it easier to deal with embarrassment or nervous feelings.

I have another reason for getting the kids to color these drawings. It helps them to remember the names of these organs. If you just look at the drawing, the names of the parts may not stick in your mind. If you spend time coloring the parts, you have to pay atten-

scrotal sac (SKROW-tuhl SAK)
testes (TES-teez)
testicles (TES-tuh-kuhls)
pubic (PEW-bik)
anus (AY-nus)
feces (FEE-sees)
bowel (BOW-uhl)

CIRCUMCISION

Figure 2 shows a *circumcised* penis. *Circumcision* is an operation which removes the *foreskin* of the penis. The foreskin is part of the special skin covering of the penis. The operation is usually done when a baby is only a few days old.

Most males in this country have been circumcised, but there are also many who still have their foreskins. If a boy has not been circumcised, his foreskin covers most or all of the glans.

When a male baby is born, the foreskin and glans are usually attached. Sooner or later, the foreskin works itself free. By the time a boy becomes an adult, if not sooner, he can retract the foreskin. This means he can pull it back over the glans and down the shaft of the penis, as shown in Figure 3.

You may be wondering why people have their sons circumcised. Maybe you have other questions about the operation. If so, you'll find more information about circumcision in Chapter 3.

tion. You're more likely to remember their names. These are important parts of the body. It's worth a little effort to learn their names.

While everyone is coloring, we talk about slang words. People don't always use the medical names for these body parts. They sometimes use slang words.

The boys in the back row of my very first puberty class were walking dictionaries of slang. Whenever I said "penis" or "vagina" out loud, their brains would buzz and hum with dozens of slang words. It was too much for them to keep to themselves. Leaning out of their seats,

circumcised (Sir-kum-sized)
circumcision (sir-kum-SISH-un)
foreskin (FOUR-skin)

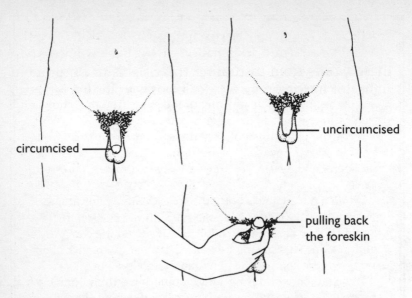

Figure 3. Circumcision

they flapped their arms, playfully punching each other. Gleefully, they whispered and hissed these so-called "dirty words" at one another. In the end, the thrill of saying these "bad" words out loud proved too much for the boys. The entire back row dissolved into fits of wild giggling. Some of them were actually rolling around on the floor. Soon, the entire class was totally out of control. "Maybe," I thought, "I'm not cut out for this line of work."

I might have given up teaching puberty classes then and there, but I had a sudden brainstorm. I turned to the blackboard and started to list all the slang words that were flying around the classroom. I encouraged the whole class to add to the list. Soon the blackboard was covered with slang words, and the class was calm enough for us to go on.

I'm not exactly sure why this works. But over the years, I've learned that it does. The best way to keep these words from disrupting the class is to bring them right out in the open. So while we're coloring, kids call out slang words and I list them on the blackboard. Here are some of them.

SOME SLANG WORDS FOR THE PENIS AND TESTICLES

PENIS			TESTICLES	
cock	peter	tool	balls	cujones
dick	dong	frankfurter	nuts	things
prick	dingus	thing	eggs	bangers
schlong	dork	pecker	rocks	hangers
wee-wee	meat	dinky	jewels	stones
wanger	pisser	penie	cubes	seeds

After we've listed them on the board, the class talks about these slang words. We discuss which words we'd use with a friend, with a doctor, or with our moms. We also talk about people's reactions to slang words. Some people object to these words. They may get upset if they hear you using them. You may or may not care about upsetting people in this way. But you should at least be aware that many people find slang words offensive.

THE FEMALE SEX ORGANS

When everyone finishes coloring the male sex organs, they color the female sex organs. The sex organs on the outside of a woman's body are called the *vulva*. The vulva has several parts. At the top is a pad of fatty tissue called the *mons*. Wiry, curly *pubic hair* covers the mons in

mons (MONZ)

grown women. I tell the class to color the mons and the pubic hair red.

Next, we move toward the bottom of the mons. There it divides into two folds of skin called the *outer lips.* I suggest blue polka dots for the outer lips. Between the outer lips lie the two *inner lips.* You might try red stripes for the inner lips.

The inner lips join at the top. The folds of skin where the lips join form a sort of hood. In Figure 2, you can see the tip of the *clitoris* peeking out from under this hood. The rest of the clitoris lies under the skin where you can't see it. Color the tip of the clitoris blue.

Straight down from the clitoris is the *urinary* opening. This is where urine leaves a woman's body. I tell the class to circle it with red.

Below the urinary opening is the *vaginal* opening. It leads to the *vagina* inside the body. The vagina connects the outside of the body to the sex organs inside a woman's body. I suggest circling the vaginal opening with blue. (People often use the word *vagina,* when they should say *vulva.* The vagina is inside the body. *Vulva* is the correct term for the sex organs on the outside of the female body.)

Finally, we come to the *anus.* Color it anyway you like.

While they're coloring the female genitals, we also make a list of slang words for these parts of a woman's body.

clitoris (KLIT-or-iss)
vaginal (VAJ-in-uhl)

SOME SLANG WORDS FOR THE CLITORIS, VULVA, AND VAGINA

CLITORIS	VULVA AND VAGINA		
clit	pussy	box	snatch
bud	cunt	beaver	poontang
pea	muff	honeypot	pudie
man in the boat	stuff	hole	slit
spot	quim	thing	twat

By the time they've colored the sex organs and made lists of slang words, everyone has giggled off a good deal of nervous energy and embarrassment. They've also gotten a good idea of where these body parts are. This helps in understanding how babies are made.

SEXUAL INTERCOURSE

Sexual intercourse between a male and a female can make a baby. When a male and female have intercourse, the penis fits inside the vagina. As soon as I tell my class this, they always have two questions right off the bat. First, they want to know *how* a penis can get inside a vagina.

I begin my answer by explaining about *erections*. Sometimes, the penis gets stiff and hard and sticks out from the body at an angle. (See Figure 4.) This is called *having an erection*. Males of all ages, even babies, have erections. An erection can happen when a male is having sexual feelings and at other times, too.

During an erection the tissue inside the penis fills with blood. This tissue has millions of tiny spaces. Usually, the spaces are empty and the penis is limp and soft. When a male has an erection, these spaces fill with so

erections (ih-REK-shuns)

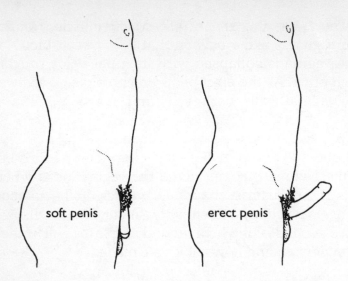

Figure 4. Erection

much blood that the tissue becomes stiff and hard. The penis swells, becomes erect, and stands out from the body. Some people call an erection a "boner" or a "hard-on." The penis can get so stiff and hard it feels like there's a bone in there. There isn't any bone, though, just blood-filled tissue.

If a couple wants to have intercourse, they get close enough together for the erect penis to be able to enter the vagina. They press their bodies together and move so the penis slides back and forth in the vagina, giving them sexual pleasure.

You might think it would be difficult for the penis to enter the vagina. Afterall, the vaginal opening isn't very large. However, the vaginal opening is *very* elastic and can stretch to many times its usual size. In fact, the vaginal opening is so elastic that when a woman gives birth, it can stretch enough to allow a baby to pass through.

The vagina is a tube of soft, pliable muscle. Normally the vagina is like a balloon that hasn't been blown up. The vagina is collapsed with its inner walls touching each other. As the erect penis enters, it pushes between the vaginal walls, parting them. The soft pliable walls mold around the erect penis for a perfect fit.

When a male is sexually excited ("turned on"), he produces a drop or two of fluid from the tip of his erect penis. Fluid also comes out of the vaginal walls when a female is sexually excited. This "wetness" helps the penis enter the vagina comfortably. Once the class understands *how* males and females have sexual intercourse, the next question is *why*.

People have sexual intercourse for many reasons. It is a special way of being close with another person. It can also feel very good. Some kids in my class find this hard to believe. But the sex organs have many nerve endings. These nerve endings send messages to pleasure centers in our brains. Stroking these parts of our bodies or rubbing them in the right ways can give us good feelings all over our bodies.

Another reason men and women have sexual intercourse is to make a baby. But babies don't start to grow every time a male and a female have intercourse, just sometimes.

Making Babies

To make a baby an *ovum* from the female and a *sperm* from the male must come together. This can happen as a result of sexual intercourse.

ovum (OH-vum)
sperm (SPURM)

Sometimes a woman's ovum is called her "egg," and a man's sperm is called his "seed." These terms confuse some of the boys and girls in my class. To them, seeds are what we plant in the ground to grow flowers or vegetables. And, eggs are what chickens lay. But, an ovum and a sperm are not like these kinds of eggs and seeds.

For starters, an ovum is much smaller than the eggs we cook for breakfast. In fact, it is smaller than the smallest dot you could make with the tip of even the sharpest pencil. A sperm is even smaller.

You could think of a sperm as half a seed and an ovum as the other half. When these two halves come together, a human baby begins to grow. Actually, the sperm and the ovum are cells. Our bodies are made of billions and billions of cells. There are many different types of cells. But the ovum and the sperm are the only kind of cells that can join together to make a single cell. From this single cell, a baby grows.

Sperm and Ejaculation

Sperm are made in the testicles, the two egg-shaped organs inside the scrotum. They are stored in hollow tubes called sperm *ducts*. A boy's testicles begin making sperm during puberty. They usually continue making new sperm every day for the rest of his life.

When he's having sex, a male may *ejaculate*. During ejaculation, muscles in the sex organs contract. These contractions pump sperm up into the main part of the body. There, they mix with other fluids. This mixture is a creamy, white fluid called *semen*. Muscle contractions

ducts (DUKTS)
ejaculate (ih-JACK-you-late)
semen (SEE-mun)

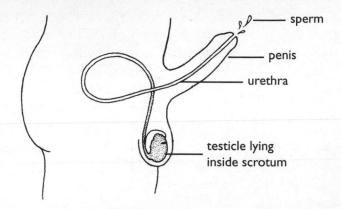

Figure 5. Ejaculation. Sperm are made in the testicles. When a man ejaculates, the sperm travel through the urethra and come out the opening in the glans.

pump the semen through the *urethra*, the hollow tube that runs the length of the penis. The semen then spurts out the opening in the tip of the penis. (See Figure 5.)

On the average, less than a teaspoon of semen comes out of the penis during an ejaculation. This small amount of semen contains millions of sperm! During sex, a male may ejaculate between 300 and 500 million sperm into the female's vagina. Some of these sperm make their way to the top of the vagina. There, they enter a tiny tunnel that leads into the *uterus* or *womb*. (See Figure 6.) The uterus is the place inside a woman's body where a baby develops.

urethra (you-REE-thruh)
uterus (YOU-ter-us)
womb (WOOM) rhymes with room

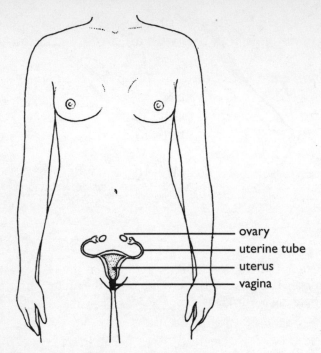

ovary
uterine tube
uterus
vagina

Figure 6. Sex Organs Inside a Woman's Body

Some of the sperm then swim to the top of the uterus and into one of the two uterine tubes. Many sperm never make it as far as the uterus. They get lost in the vagina or the tiny tunnel. Other sperm get lost in the uterus. The sperm that get lost and don't make it are eventually dissolved by the woman's body.

Of the millions of sperm ejaculated into the vagina, only a few make it to the top of the uterus and from there into the *uterine* tubes. There are two uterine tubes that connect to the upper part of the uterus on either

uterine (YOU-ter-in)

side. Here, inside one of these tubes, the sperm may meet and join together with an ovum.

Ovum and Ovulation

A girl is born with hundreds of thousands of *ova*. (Ova is the plural form of ovum. If you're talking about more than one ovum, you say ova.) Ova are stored in two organs called *ovaries*.

A young girl's ova are not mature. The first ovum doesn't ripen until she is well into puberty. A grown woman usually produces a ripe ovum from one of her ovaries about once a month. When it is fully mature, the ripe ovum pops off the *ovary*. This release of the ripe ovum from the ovary is called *ovulation*. (See Figure 7.)

After it pops off the ovary, the ovum enters one of the uterine tubes. The ends of the uterine tube reach out and sweep the ovum into the tube. Tiny hairs inside the tube wave back and forth. Slowly, their gentle waving helps move the ovum through the tube.

Fertilization, Pregnancy, and Birth

As the ovum travels through the tube, it may meet some sperm. If so, one of the sperm may enter the ovum. This joining of an ovum and a sperm is called *fertilization*.

The ovum can be *fertilized* by a sperm only during the first twenty-four hours after it leaves the ovary. But,

ova (OH-vuh)
ovaries (OH-vuh-reez)
ovary (OH-vuh-ree)
ovulation (ahv-you-LAY-shun)
fertilization (fur-till-eye-ZAY-shun)
fertilized (FUR-till-eye-zed)

sperm can stay alive inside the female body for up to five days. This means fertilization is possible if a male and female have sex on the day of ovulation or on any of the five days before ovulation. Most times, the ovum travels through the uterine tube into the uterus without meeting a sperm. A few days after it reaches the uterus, the unfertilized ovum breaks down.

If the ovum has been fertilized, it doesn't break down. Once it gets to the uterus, it plants itself there, and, over the next nine months, it grows into a baby.

The uterus is a hollow organ. In a grown woman, the uterus is normally the size of a pear. But, the thick, muscular walls of the uterus are very elastic. This allows the uterus to expand during pregnancy. (See Figure 8.)

When the baby is ready to come out, the mother's uterus begins to contract. The tiny tunnel connecting the uterus to the vagina stretches open. Powerful contrac-

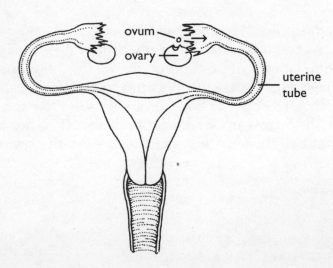

Figure 7. Ovulation

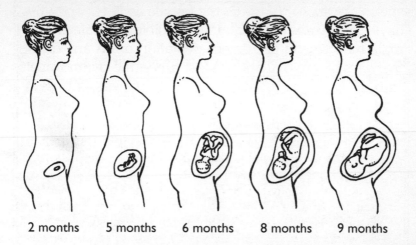

| 2 months | 5 months | 6 months | 8 months | 9 months |

Figure 8. Pregnancy. A fetilized ovum plants itself on the inside wall of the uterus, and over the next nine months, it develops into a baby.

tions push the baby out of the uterus and into the vagina. The contractions continue. The baby is pushed through the vagina, then out the vaginal opening, and into the world. Hello baby!

EVERYTHING YOU EVER WANTED TO KNOW...

If you're like the boys in our classes and workshops, you have lots of questions about what's happening to your body. It isn't always easy to ask these questions. We may feel too embarrassed. We may think our questions are too dumb. We may be afraid that everyone else already knows the answers. Maybe they'll laugh at us. Maybe they'll think we're stupid or "out of it."

If you've ever felt like this, you're not alone. In my classes, we play a game called "Everything You Ever Wanted To Know About Puberty And Sex But Were

TWINS, SIAMESE TWINS, TRIPLETS . . .

As soon as I explain about fertilization, hands shoot up all around the classroom.

"What if more than one sperm fertilizes the egg? Will the woman have twins?"

I explain that it's only possible for one sperm to enter an ovum and fertilize it. The instant a sperm begins to enter, the ovum goes through chemical changes. These changes make it impossible for another sperm to enter.

But that's usually just the beginning of the questions. Although, it would take another whole book to answer all the questions. Here are some basic facts to help satisfy your curiosity.

• *Fraternal* twins are one of the two types of twins. (See Figure 9.) Fraternal twins happen when there are two ova, each fertilized by a different sperm. Usually a woman's ovary produces only one ripe ovum at a time, but once in a while the ovary produces two ripe ova at the same time. Each of these ova could then be fertilized by a different sperm. If both fertilized ova plant themselves in the lining of the uterus, the woman will be pregnant with fraternal twins. Such twins may not look alike. They may not even be the same sex.

• *Identical* twins develop from a single fertilized ovum that splits in two. (See Figure 10.) The splitting happens soon after the fertilization. No one knows why. Because identical twins come from the same ovum and sperm, they look alike. They are always the same sex.

• When twins are born, one baby comes out first. The other baby usually comes out a few minutes later. Sometimes more time passes before the second twin is born. There have even been cases when a whole day passed between the births of the first and second twin.

• It is possible for a woman to give birth to fraternal twins who have two different fathers. For this to happen, the

fraternal (fruh-TURN-uhl)
identical (eye-DEN-ti-kuhl)

woman would have to have sex with two different men right around the time she ovulates.

• *Siamese* twins are identical twins who are born with their bodies attached to each other in some way. For some unknown reason, the fertilized ovum doesn't split completely. The babies develop with parts of their bodies joined together.

Identical twins are pretty rare. Siamese twins are much rarer. Siamese twins may be joined in a number of ways. If they are joined at the feet, the shoulders, or the arms, an operation can separate the babies. In other cases, it's more difficult to separate them. They may be joined in such a way that cutting them apart would kill one or both. For instance, the bodies may be joined at the chest and share one heart. Some parents decide to have the operation done even if one baby may die. Other parents decide against the operation. If they aren't separated, the twins spend their lives attached.

• Triplets (three babies), quadruplets (four), quintuplets (five), sextuplets (six), septuplets (seven), and octuplets (eight) happen even less often than twins. When more than three babies are born at one time, the chance of all the babies surviving is low. Because there are so many of them, they're much smaller than normal babies and are born before they develop fully. As far as we know, the largest number of babies born at one time is twelve. But some of them died. There was a case in Iowa where a woman gave birth to seven babies, all of whom survived. Not too long after that, eight live babies were born to a couple in Texas, but one of them died shortly after birth.

Women who give birth to several or more babies at one time are usually taking special medicines to get pregnant. Because these women have had problems getting pregnant in the past, their doctors put them on drugs to stimulate the ovaries. But, such drugs often stimulate the ovaries too much, so that several ripe ova are released at the same time.

Siamese (sigh-UH-meez)

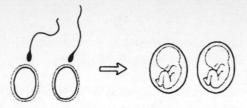

Figure 9. Fraternal Twins. Fraternal twins happen when a woman produces two ripe ova, each of which is fertilized by a different sperm.

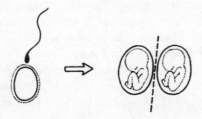

Figure 10. Identical Twins. Identical twins happen when, after fertilization, the ovum splits into two. Identical twins look alike and are always of the same sex.

Afraid To Ask." We pass out slips of paper at the beginning of class. The kids can write their questions and put the slips in a special box. They don't have to sign their names. I am the only one who gets to see the question slips. The box is locked and it stays in the classroom. Kids can write down questions any time and put them in the box. At the end of class, I open the question box. I read the questions out loud and do my best to answer them. (If I don't know the answer, I say so. Then I make a point of trying to find the answer before the next class.)

Here are some questions from our question box:

What's the largest penis measurement in the world? Can a penis be too small?

When will I grow a beard and start to look like my dad?

Why do you sometimes get a hard-on when you're not even thinking about sex?

I have a line that runs down the back of my balls. Is this normal?

Is there something wrong if you have one testicle lower than the other?

How tall will I be?

Is there a way to make your penis bigger?

Which way should your penis curve when it's hard?

How old do you have to be to have a wet dream?

I don't have much hair on my balls. Is something wrong?

Can a boy grow breasts?

Is it okay to jack off?

What if you masturbate and only clear stuff comes out?

I have little white bumps on my penis. Does that mean I have some kind of disease?

My balls are huge, but my penis is tiny. What is wrong?

What's the best stuff for zits?

I have a pain in my penis and some white stuff that looks like milk has been coming out. What's wrong?

What's the right age for starting puberty?

How can you tell if you're gay?

If you ejaculate too often, can this hurt you? Will you run out of sperm?

Is it true that girls bleed once a month after they go through puberty?

How long does puberty take?

If you like a girl, how should you act so she'll like you?

READING THIS BOOK

This book answers these and other questions from our class question box, our workshops, and our readers. You may want to read this book with your parents, with a friend, or by yourself. You may want to read it straight through from beginning to end. Or, perhaps, you'll jump around, reading a chapter here and there. However you read this book, we hope that you'll enjoy it. We hope, too, that you'll learn as much from reading it as we did from writing it.

CHAPTER 2

Beginning Changes and the Stages of Puberty

Growing vegetables is one of my hobbies. I like to pretend that it saves me lots of money. The truth is I spend a small fortune on gardening books, fertilizers, and netting to keep birds from eating it all. In the end, each pound of vegetables from my garden winds up costing me about fifty bucks.

You may be asking yourself what my vegetable garden has to do with boys and puberty. The answer is, nothing at all. Except for this: each of the plants in my garden has its own way and time of growing. I can take two seeds from the same package and plant them next to each other in my garden. I give them both the same amount of water. They both get the same amount of sunshine. Yet one seedling pops out of the ground and is three or four inches high before the other has even broken through the soil. Boys, too, have their own way and time of growing.

Take the boys in Figure 11. Both boys are twelve years old. Both are completely healthy, normal, and regular in every way. One boy is well into puberty. His sex organs have begun to grow and develop, and he has a lot of

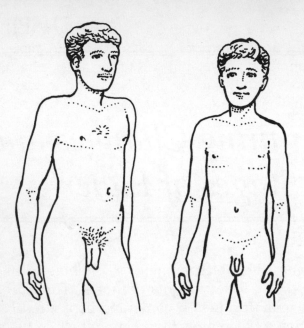

Figure 11. Two Twelve-Year-Olds. Both these boys are twelve. One has already developed quite a bit. The other is just beginning puberty.

pubic hair. He is already quite tall and has developed bigger muscles, as well as some body and facial hair. The other boy hasn't developed nearly so much. He is just beginning puberty. These boys have different timetables and are at different stages of development. But, both boys are developing normally, at the right age and time for their own bodies.

STARTING EARLY, STARTING LATE

Puberty starts at different ages for different boys. Some boys start to develop when they're only nine. Others don't start until they're fourteen, or even fifteen years old.

Why do some boys start early, at a young age, and others not until they're older? The complete answer to this question isn't in yet, but part of the answer has to do with a boy's family background. Boys tend to take after their dads and the males in their dad's family. If your dad and his male relatives started puberty at an early age, you probably will, too. If they were late-starters, it's likely you'll be a late starter, too.

This is not a hard and fast rule. A boy may differ from his dad and the male relatives. For instance, a boy from a family of late starters could begin puberty at the average age or even earlier. Also, your male relatives may not have a common pattern. They may be a mix of average, early, and late starters. But males from the same family are often alike in this way, so, it's worth asking your relatives when they started to develop.

DEVELOPING QUICKLY, DEVELOPING SLOWLY

Meanwhile, back in my garden . . . The first seedlings to pop up always stay a step ahead of the other seedlings. They quickly develop into fully grown plants. Many people assume it works the same way with boys going through puberty. They figure the boys who start early will develop faster than other boys. But that's not always the case.

Some early starters *do* develop very quickly. They begin puberty at a young age and quickly develop mature, adult bodies. Other early-starters develop at the average rate, and still others develop slowly. The same is true for boys who are late starters and for boys who start at the average age. The age at which a boy starts puberty doesn't tell us how quickly (or slowly) he will develop.

Most boys take three or four years to go through puberty. But some boys take five years or more to mature, while others take less than two years. Again, the amount of time it takes for a boy to go through puberty is *not related* to the age at which he starts.

FIRST CHANGES

For most boys, the first outward sign of puberty comes when their testicles and scrotum begin to develop. During childhood, the sex organs don't grow very much. During puberty, the sex organs go through a growth spurt. They start to grow larger at a much faster rate than during childhood.

The scrotum and testicles are the first to start developing. The testicles enlarge. The scrotum gets longer and the testicles hang lower. The skin of the scrotum reddens or gets darker in color. It also gets thinner and the scrotum gets looser. Later, the penis starts to develop, growing longer and then wider. At some point, pubic hair starts to grow on the genitals.

Although the growth of the testicles and scrotum is usually the first puberty change, many boys don't notice this change. The testicles are pretty small before puberty. Even when they do start growing, they are still pretty small at first. It can be difficult to tell if your testicles have started growing. Understanding how doctors measure testicle size may help you tell if your testicles have started growing.

Measuring Testicle Size

Doctors measure testicle size with a tool called an *orchidometer*. It is a set of egg-shaped wooden or plastic ovals. The ovals are strung together on a cord according

orchidometer (OR-kih-DOM-uh-ter)

to size. Figure 12 is a life-size drawing of an orchidometer.

The doctor holds the orchidometer in one hand and the patient's testicle in the other. The doctor slides the ovals through one hand, comparing their size to that of the testicle in the other hand. The doctor "sizes" the testicle by choosing the oval that is closest to the testicle in size and reading the number printed on the oval.

The number on the oval shows its size in terms of its volume (how much it can hold). The volume is measured in milliliters (ml for short). The oval marked 1 has a volume of 1 ml. This is about one-fifth of a teaspoon. The largest oval, the one marked 25, has a volume of 25 ml. This is about five teaspoons.

You probably don't have a spare orchidometer lying around the house, but you can get a rough idea of your size by comparing your testicles to the drawing of the orchidometer in this book. Which oval are you closest to?

Size each testicle. Don't worry if one is a little larger than the other. This is perfectly normal. In grown men, the right testicle is usually (but not always) larger than the left testicle. However, the left testicle usually hangs lower. If your testicles are 4 ml or more in size, this is a pretty reliable sign that puberty has started. If your testicles are 3 ml or less in size, you probably haven't started puberty.

Pubic Hair

During puberty you also begin to grow pubic hair. Often, this is the first change that boys themselves notice. As we said, testicle growth comes first, but as we also said testicle growth can be hard to detect. Some boys begin to grow pubic hair at about the same time their testicles start to grow. Other boys don't grow

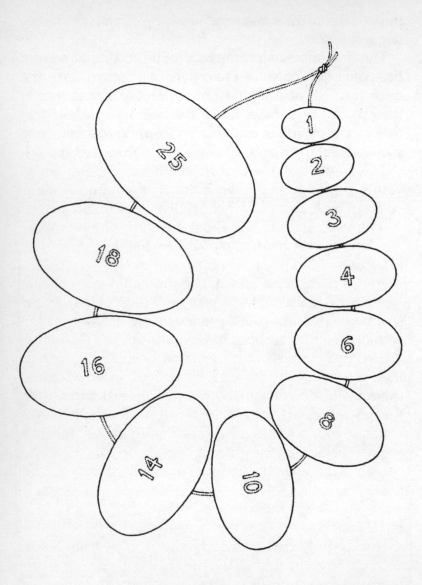

Figure 12. Orchidometer. This drawing is life size.

pubic hair until sometime after their testicles have begun to grow.

The first pubic hairs are not usually very dark in color or very curly. There aren't very many of them. The first hairs usually begin growing in the area where the penis joins the body. As puberty continues, the pubic hairs get darker and curlier. There will also be more of them. They grow above the penis, on the lower abdomen (belly),

HANGING LOW, KEEPING COOL

Did you ever wonder why the scrotum and testicles hang down, outside and away from the main part of your body? One boy in my class put the question this way:

Why do they dangle down there like that where they can get hit and knocked around? Why aren't they tucked up inside your body where they'd be safe?

Andy, age 11

It's a good question, and there's a good answer. Sperm, the male reproductive cells, are made in the testicles. To make sperm, your testicles have to be at just the right temperature. This temperature is a little lower than normal body temperature. Up inside your body, it's too warm for your testicles to make sperm. Instead, they hang down in the scrotum, away from the body, where it's cooler. Air circulates around the scrotum helping to keep the testicles cool.

The scrotum does its best to keep the testicles at just the right temperature. In cold weather or when you jump into a cold pool, the scrotum tightens up. This brings your testicles closer to your body for extra warmth. In hot weather, after a hot bath, or when you have a fever, the scrotum relaxes and hangs lower. Your testicles are further from your body so they stay cooler.

and spread out toward the thighs. They may also grow on the scrotum or near the anus. In adult men, pubic hair grows in an upside-down triangle pattern on the lower part of the belly. It may also grow up toward the belly button and out to the thighs.

Your pubic hair is usually the same color as the hair on your head, but it can be lighter or darker. The amount of pubic hair depends on ethnic, racial, and family background. For example, Chinese and Japanese are likely to have less pubic hair and to develop it later in puberty than Europeans or Africans.

Some of the boys and men we talked to were a bit worried when they started to grow pubic hair. Here is what some of them had to say:

> It looked like I was getting all these pimples on the skin around my cock.
>
> *Jim, age 16*

> There were little raised bumps, and I thought I had some kind of disease.
>
> *Phil, age 24*

> First I got these tiny, kind of whitish, raised spots. I was scared to say anything. I just waited. Then I noticed these fuzzy hairs growing out.
>
> *Bill, age 17*

When pubic hair starts to grow, little bumps often appear on the surface of the skin. They may look like pimples. These bumps are caused by the tiny pubic hairs pushing through the skin. Soon, little hairs begin to poke through the surface of the bumps. If you don't know what is going on, you may be worried. But it is a perfectly normal part of growing up. It is not anything to worry about.

You may notice that you have other little bumps or dots on the skin of the penis and scrotum—ones that do not grow little hairs. These are oil and perspiration (sweat) glands. They make small amounts of oil and perspiration. You may also notice that the skin in this area feels moister or smells a bit different. The oil and sweat glands that become active during puberty cause these changes. They are a normal and natural part of growing up, another sign that you are becoming a man.

THE STAGES OF PUBERTY

Doctors divide the growth and development of the genital organs into five stages. These stages are shown in Figure 13. Doctors also divide pubic hair growth into five stages. Figure 14 shows the stages of pubic hair growth. Read the descriptions of these stages in this section. Then, compare your body to the drawings of these stages. What stages are you in?

By the way, genital and pubic hair stages don't always match. You may be in one stage of genital development and in a different stage of pubic hair growth. For example, you might be in Stage 2 of genital development and Stage 1 of pubic hair growth. So, don't worry if your genital and pubic hair stages don't match. It's perfectly normal!

When genital and pubic hair are at different stages, pubic hair growth usually, but not always, lags behind genital development. In other words, it's more likely for a boy to be in Genital Stage 3 and Pubic Hair Stage 2 than the other way around.

When stages don't match, there's usually not a big difference between the two types of development. Usually, pubic hair doesn't lag behind genital growth by more than one to two stages. This isn't always the case, though. Sometimes one type of development is quite a bit slower than the other. For example, sometimes a boy is in Stage 4 of genital development before he grows his first pubic hair. This, too, is perfectly normal.

Five Stages of Genital Growth and Development

The five stages of sex organ growth and development are shown in Figure 13 and described below.

Stage 1: Childhood

Stage 1 is childhood, before puberty begins. Your sex organs do not change very much during this stage. As the rest of your body grows, the penis, scrotum, and testicles grow a little bit larger, too, but not by very much. What growth there is takes place very slowly. The testicles are usually less than 3 ml in size.

You won't have any pubic hair yet. Boys usually don't grow pubic hair until Stage 2 or later.

Stage 2: Testicles and Scrotum Enlarge

Stage 2 is the beginning of puberty. A boy reaches Stage 2 when his testicles and scrotum begin to enlarge. During childhood, these sex organs grow very slowly. When puberty hits, they start growing at a much faster rate. If your testicles are 4 ml or larger in size, you have probably reached Stage 2 and started puberty.

The penis itself doesn't get much larger in this stage. The biggest change is in the size of the testicles and scrotum. As the testicles grow larger, the scrotum gets longer. The testicles and scrotum hang lower. The skin of the scrotum gets thinner and looser. The scrotum is more baggy and wrinkled. The testicles no longer fill the scrotal sac. The skin of the scrotum has a new "feel" to it.

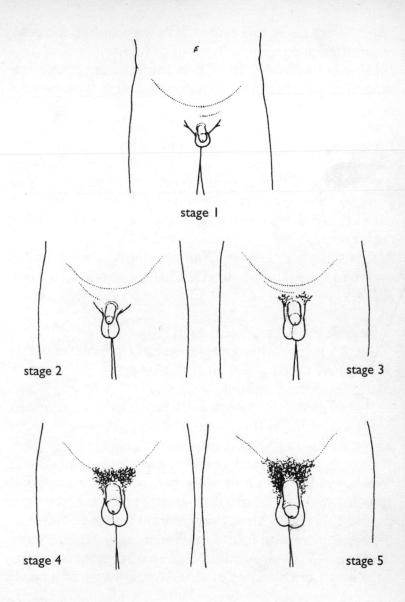

Figure 13. Five Stages of Genital Development

The color changes too. The skin of the scrotum reddens or gets darker in color.

Most boys develop their first pubic hairs during this stage. But many boys don't develop their first pubic hair until Stage 3 or later.

Boys typically reach Stage 2 when they're ten to twelve years old, but there are many boys who start this stage when they are only nine. There are also many who don't start until they're thirteen or nearly fourteen. There are also some perfectly normal and healthy boys who get to Stage 2 even earlier than the age of eight or later than age fourteen.

This stage may last anywhere from just a few months or for more than two years. On the average, it lasts about a year.

Stage 3: The Penis Grows Longer

Stage 3 begins when the penis starts to grow longer. It doesn't get much wider during this stage. The biggest change is in the length of the penis.

The skin of the penis and scrotum continues to deepen in color in this stage. The scrotum and testicles also continue to grow during this stage.

If your pubic hair didn't start growing during Stage 2, you may notice your first pubic hairs during this stage. If you already have pubic hair, it may get darker and curlier during this stage. Most boys reach this stage between the ages of ten and fourteen. The average age for starting Stage 4 is twelve or thirteen. This stage usually lasts anywhere from a couple of months to a year and a half.

Stage 4: The Penis Grows Wider

In Stage 4, the penis grows wider and the glans becomes more developed. The penis also continues to grow longer, but the major changes are in its width and in the glans. The skin of the scrotum and penis continues to darken in color. The testicles continue to grow and the scrotum hangs lower. Most boys have pubic hair when they start Stage 4. But, there are some who don't develop pubic hair until they reach this stage.

Boys typically start Stage 4 when they are thirteen or fourteen years old. But many boys are only eleven or twelve when they start this stage. There are also many boys who are fifteen, sixteen, or seventeen before they reach this stage. Here again, there are a few perfectly healthy normal boys who fall outside these age ranges. This stage usually lasts anywhere from one half to two years.

Stage 5: Adult Stage

This is the final, mature stage. The testicles are fully grown. They are usually about 1 ¾ inches long and between 14 and 27 ml. in size. The scrotum is also fully developed. The skin of the scrotum and penis has gotten even deeper in color.

The penis is now fully developed. As with other parts of the body, the size of the penis varies from one person to the next. We'll talk more about penis size in Chapter 3.

Boys typically reach Stage 5 when they are fourteen to sixteen years old. But, some boys reach this stage when they're only twelve or thirteen and others not until they're older than sixteen. As with the other stages, some normal boys will fall outside the age ranges given here.

Five Stages of Pubic Hair Growth

As we said earlier, doctors divide pubic hair growth in five stages. The stages are shown in Figure 14 and described below.

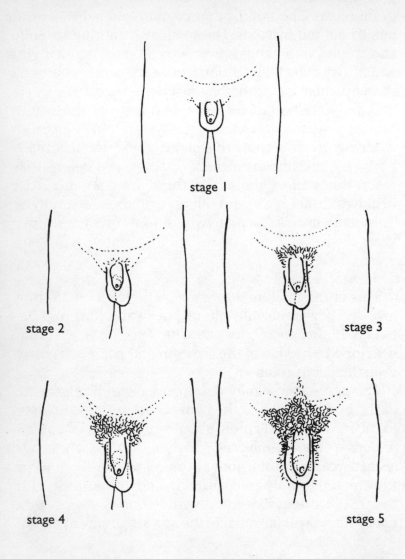

Figure 14. Five Stages of Pubic Hair Growth

Stage 1: Childhood

This is the childhood, or prepuberty, stage. There is no pubic hair. You may have some hair on your lower belly and around your genitals in this stage. If so, it's the light, downy type of hair like peach fuzz that grows on the belly and elsewhere on the body. This childhood hair is short, fine, and soft. It has little color and is not pubic hair.

Stage 2: First Pubic Hairs Appear

This stage starts when the first pubic hairs appear. The first hairs are straight or a only a bit curly. They have some color, but not much. They are longer than the childhood hairs seen in Stage 1. These first hairs usually grow around the base of the penis, where it joins the body. There may be just a few of them. You may have to look very closely to see them. Look in the area where the penis joins the body.

Stage 3: Growth Continues

In this stage, the pubic hair is curlier, coarser, and darker in color. It covers a wider area and there is more of it, but still not a lot. The hair growth may extend to the scrotum.

Stage 4: Almost Adult

The pubic hairs are now as dark, curly, and coarse as adult pubic hair. There is a good deal more pubic hair than there was in Stage 3. The hair growth may have a triangle pattern, but it doesn't extend to the thighs. It doesn't cover as wide an area as it will in Stage 5.

Stage 5: Adult

This is the adult stage. The pubic hair is coarse and curly. It now reaches to the edge of the thigh on either side. It usually grows in an upside-down triangle pattern, extending up toward the belly button and out onto the thighs.

Some boys—in particular, Chinese boys, and other Asians as well—do not develop pubic hair beyond Stage 3 or 4. For them, these stages are the adult stage of development.

FEELINGS ABOUT PUBERTY

The kids in my second and third grade classes usually haven't started puberty yet. They are usually excited and can hardly wait for puberty to begin. They don't all feel this way, though. One third grader put it like this:

> Ugh! I don't want my penis to get all big and hairy and ugly looking!
>
> *Jonathan, age 8*

In my classes for older kids, most have started puberty or will soon. Like the younger kids, they are usually excited. They are pleased and proud when they notice their bodies starting to change. As one boy said:

> It's a "Hey, whoopee, I'm finally growing up!" kind of feeling.
>
> *Jose, age 12*

The older kids usually have other feelings along with the excited, proud feelings. This is totally normal. Almost everyone has some doubts. One boy put it this way:

> I was taking a bath . . . and I saw that I had some pubic hairs. I guess my penis and balls had been getting bigger all along . . . I really realized I was changing. I felt grown up and I was really jazzed about it. Then, two seconds later, I had this really scared feeling . . . "Oh, no, I'm not ready for this."
>
> *James, age 11*

Many of the men and boys we talked to had these "I'm-not-ready" feelings. If you feel this way, it helps to remember that it's perfectly normal.

Some boys get to feeling down because their bodies are slow to develop. They're eager to have mature, muscular bodies. Their classmates may be developing while they still look "like little kids."

Some men remembered how difficult it was to be a late starter.

> I didn't go through puberty until I was sixteen. It really bothered me when I was in situations where other boys could see that I hadn't started yet. I was always embarrassed in gym class and I always tried to hide my body.
>
> *Jim, age 47*

> I was a late starter, too. It seemed like all the other guys had really developed bodies and hair all over the place, and here I was still a skinny, little kid. Once it started, though, I really developed fast. My whole attitude was, "Thank God! At last it's happening to me." For a while there, I was thinking it would never happen and that maybe I was some kind of freak or maybe I was sick or there was something wrong. But, finally, I started to develop, too.
>
> *Glenn, age 42*

If you're worried that puberty is never going to happen to you, take a look around. How many adults do you know who've never gone through puberty? None, right? We all go through puberty sooner or later. Before too long your body will change and you'll catch up to the other kids. Then you'll wonder what all the fuss was about! It's not just late starters who feel embarrassed. One man remembered how he felt about being an early starter:

> I developed at a very early age. I was really proud, but also embarrassed because I looked so different from the other kids.

It's hard at that age to be different. You want to be just like the other guys and not stand out.

Pete, age 26

It *is* difficult to be different. But try to remember there is no "right" age for everyone. Your body is developing at the age that's right for you.

AM I NORMAL?

Seems like everyone asks this question at some point during puberty. The answer is almost always "yes." But, though they are not common, there are medical problems that can cause puberty to start either too early or too late.

It's not always easy to know what's "too early" or "too late." As you've learned in this chapter, boys start puberty at very different ages. Some perfectly normal, healthy boys notice the first signs of puberty when they are only eight or even younger. Other perfectly normal, healthy boys don't start puberty until they're fourteen or older.

Doctors usually recommend that boys who start puberty before the age of eight and a half to nine should have a medical checkup. In other words, a boy should see a doctor if his testicles or penis begin to develop, if he grows pubic hair or if he develops any other sign of puberty before he's nine.

Doctors also recommend that boys who haven't started puberty by their fourteenth or fifteenth birthday should have a medical checkup. In other words, a boy whose sex organs have not begun to develop and has no pubic hair by his fourteenth or fifteenth birthday, should see a doctor.

It's important to remember that starting before the age of nine or after the age of fourteen or fifteen does not always mean there is something wrong. However, when there is something wrong, the problem can be treated by a doctor, so the boy can develop normally.

Sometimes puberty seems to go very slowly. The changes in our bodies may be so slight that we wonder if we're really growing at all. Or, we wonder if the whole thing has stopped altogether. If you've started puberty, but your growth isn't as fast as you'd like, hang in there. You are growing and will wind up with a mature, adult body.

Of course, if you feel that something isn't right with the way your body is developing, you can see a doctor at any time. If it turns out that you do have a medical problem, you'll have caught it that much earlier. If you don't have a problem, you'll feel better knowing that there's nothing wrong.

CHAPTER 3

An Owner's Guide to the Sex Organs: What's Normal? What's Not?

Chapter 2 explained how the sex organs on the outside of the body change during puberty. Boys are naturally curious about these changes. Younger boys often study their bodies carefully, looking for the first signs of change. Even boys who haven't been on the lookout for these changes start paying close attention once their sex organs start to grow.

Once they start paying more attention to their bodies, boys often have questions or concerns about their sex organs. Perhaps they notice something they never noticed before. Or, maybe, it's something they noticed but never really thought about before. Whatever the reason, boys your age often have questions and concerns about the size, shape, or appearance of their sex organs.

This chapter is an "owner's guide" to the sex organs on the outside of the male body. Like other parts of the body, the penis and scrotum look different in different people. There's a lot of individual variation in the way these sex organs look. The guide explains these differences, so you'll know what's normal and what's not.

PENIS SIZE

Penis size is the biggest concern. (No pun intended.) If you've worried about the size of yours, you're not alone! This topic comes up over and over again in our question boxes and in readers' letters. In fact, we get more questions about penis size than all other topics combined.

One of the earliest scientific reports on penis size dates back to 1879. Its author, Dr. W. Krause, reported that "in most cases" the erect penis is just under 8 ¼ inches long. Maybe the whole problem of men thinking their penises are too small can be traced back to this report. Or maybe not. But the fact is, Dr. K. was off by more than two inches. Most guys will fall short of the mark trying to measure up to 8 ¼ inches. Only one in a hundred grown men has an erect penis that long!

The Long and Short of It

We'll get to the more up-to-date, scientific reports of penis size in just a page or two. First, though, we want to clear up a couple of size issues.

Many boys think their penises are too small. They look around the locker room and everyone's penis seems bigger than theirs. But comparing sizes this way can be very misleading.

There's a lot of variation in the size of the soft penis. But size differences tend to disappear when an erection appears. Penises that are on the small side when soft tend to grow more during an erection. Penises that are larger than most when soft tend to grow less. If your penis is on the small side when soft, this doesn't mean it will be on the small side when erect.

It's difficult to even say what the average size of the soft penis is. That's because the size changes so much.

Being afraid, cold, or nervous can reduce blood inside the penis, making it smaller in size. The penis can shrink by as much as two inches. Being relaxed or warm increases the blood in the penis, making it larger. That's why it's difficult to say what the average size of *one* man's penis is when it's soft, much less the average of *all* men's. That's also why most scientific studies measure the size of the erect penis.

It's natural for boys to make locker room comparisons. It's natural to want to see how you measure up against the "average" penis size. But, don't forget, you're still growing. Remember what you learned in Chapter 2. The penis doesn't reach full size until Stage 5. If you're not in Stage 5 yet, you've still got a lot of growing to do. Even once you reach Stage 5, your penis may continue to grow. Many a boy is seventeen or eighteen or even older before his penis reaches its full size.

The penis doesn't really start to grow until Stage 3. The guy next to you in the gym showers may be the same age, but he may be at a very different stage of puberty. He may be in Stage 4 or 5 already. If you're still in Stage 2, of course his penis is bigger than yours. That doesn't mean yours is too small. When you get to Stage 5, your penis will probably be about the same as most other guys' penises.

The size of your erection varies, too. There may not be as much variation as there is in the size of soft penises. But erection size is affected by room temperature, how nervous you are, the time of day, recent sexual activity, the situation, and your mood.

About Average

Penis size is a very important issue with men. You would think there would be all sorts of good, scientific studies of penis size. There aren't. Not very many studies have been done. And the studies we do have may not be reliable. Some of them have too few men in them to be reliable. In other studies, volunteers measured their penis size at home, without scientific supervision. Even if the men were honest in their measurements, they may not have followed the directions properly. For instance some may have "rounded up" to the next highest number when reporting their size. Perhaps men with large penises would be more likely to volunteer for this type of study than men with small penises. If so, the "average size" reported by the study would be too big. Keep all this in mind as we tell you about the results from these studies.

The famous sex researcher, Alfred Kinsey, and his coworkers studied penis size. Thousands of volunteers were asked to measure the length of their erect penis and mail in the results. The average erect penis size from the Kinsey studies was just under 6 ¼ inches. There are some newer studies where the measuring was done by doctors or from photographs. These studies show an average erect penis length of very close to six inches. But, again, some of these studies had to rely on volunteers, which may have affected the results.

The best we can do is to tell you results based on less than perfect studies. These studies tell us that 7 out of 10 adult men have erect penises between 5 ¼ and 6 ¾ inches in length. Also, in adult men the average distance measuring around the widest part of an erect penis is a little under five inches.

Myths About Penis Size

Myths are stories or legends. Many myths are completely false. Here are some myths that people tell about penis size, along with the real facts.

MEASURING UP

In scientific studies, the length of the penis is measured along the top of the penis, from the point where it joins the body to its tip. Most men have measured theirs at least once in their lives. It's easy enough to do. All you need is a ruler, an erection, and the following directions:

When you are fully erect and standing, angle your penis so that it is perpendicular (sticks straight out) from your body. Lay the ruler along the top of your penis. Make your penis as straight as you can, so it is as flat as possible against the ruler. Press one end of the ruler into the pubic area at the base of your penis. Measure the distance to the tip of the penis.

Use a ruler, not a tape measure. A ruler is rigid and can be firmly pressed into the pad of fat that covers the pubic bone.

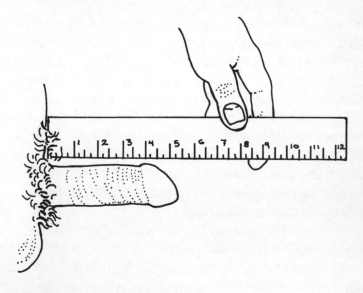

Figure 15. Measuring the Penis

Myth: Men with big penises are more masculine or macho than men with smaller penises. This myth takes various forms depending on what people consider masculine. For example, you may have heard that men who have large penises are better at sports, or that they are braver, or stronger.

Fact: It simply isn't true. The size of your penis does not have anything to do with how brave or strong or athletic you are.

Myth: Men with big penises are sexually more powerful. People say this myth in different ways, too. For example, men with big penises have a stronger sexual drive. Or, they have a larger sexual appetite. Or, they have more erections. Or, they have erections that last longer.

Fact: The size of your penis does not have anything to do with any of these things. Different men have different sexual drives. Some have erections more quickly than others. But these differences have nothing to do with their penis size.

Myth: Men with big penises make better lovers. This, too, comes in several versions. Women enjoy sex more if the man has a big penis. Women find men with big penises more attractive.

Fact: Penis size has very little to do with how much a woman enjoys sexual intercourse. A woman's pleasure in intercourse comes mostly from the stimulation she gets in the area around the clitoris. It is on the outside, rather than inside the vagina. Only the first inch or two of the vagina contains nerve endings. The upper parts of the vagina are not very sensitive. A woman's pleasure is also affected by her emotional feelings for her partner. In

Make your penis longer and thicker . . .
Erect measurements up to 12 inches or more!
Grow to your maximum potential!
Scientifically proven to work!

These claims are from ads for "penis enlargers" or "penis enlargement systems." Some of these products, like "sex drops" or "penis creams," are useless and just plain silly.

Some products are kits with weights you attach to the penis to stretch it. These kits are not only useless, but may be dangerous. In some cases, what you get is a cheap version of a medical device called a "penis pump." The device was invented for men with health problems who can't get normal erections. The pump can make the penis harder and longer. But, like an erection, the pump only makes the penis larger for a while. Once you stop the pump, you'll be your same old self again. Meanwhile, you can do serious damage to the penis with the pump.

You can't change your penis size by exercise, hypnotism, pills, creams, pumps, or other gadgets. Don't be fooled by the ads. If it sounds too good to be true, it is. Don't waste your money. These products don't work, and some of them could hurt your penis.

all these factors, penis size is of little or no importance.

There are no scientific studies to suggest that women prefer men with big penises. There *are* studies that show that women do not care about their partner's penis size.

Myth: African-American men have bigger penises than men in other racial or ethnic groups.

Fact: There may be some racial differences in penis size, but these are not very large. The average erect penis length of African-American men in Kinsey studies was one-tenth of an inch larger than the average for white men. Some studies have shown small differences between other racial and ethnic groups.

We hope this section has made you understand one basic fact. Your penis size is an indication of one thing and one thing only: the size of your penis. Your penis size has nothing to do with what kind lover, husband, athlete, or father you'll be. It has nothing to do with how macho, manly, or brave you are. Honest.

THE PENIS: CIRCUMCISED AND UNCIRCUMCISED

It's not just the size of the penis that varies from boy to boy or man to man. The appearance does too. One basic difference is circumcision. (Circumcision, remember, is the operation which removes the foreskin of the penis.) A circumcised penis looks different than one that isn't circumcised.

The penis shown in Figure 16 has been circumcised. The foreskin has been removed. You can see all of the glans, or head, of the penis. The *corona*, the rounded ridge of tissue around the bottom edge of the glans, is clearly visible.

The penis shown in Figure 17 has not been circumcised. The foreskin is intact and not retracted. It covers the corona and all but the tip of the glans. (Some foreskins are longer than the one shown here. Others are shorter. Shorter ones cover less of the glans. Longer ones cover more and may extend beyond, or "overhang," the glans.)

corona (kor-OH-nuh)

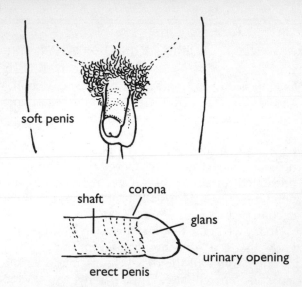

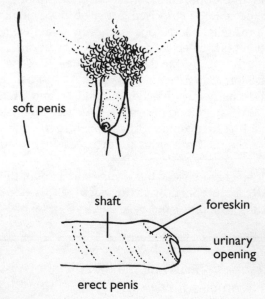

Figure 16. Circumcised Penis

Figure 17. Uncircumcised Penis. In both these drawings the foreskin is not retracted.

CIRCUMCISION—WHY?

Circumcision has long been a religious custom in the Jewish and Muslim faiths. In the mid- to late 1800s, doctors in this country and in Europe began recommending circumcision for all male babies. These doctors believed the operation was painless due to the "undeveloped" nervous system of the newborn baby. They also believed that circumcision cured or prevented certain diseases. Circumcision caught on. And, at one time, nearly all male babies born in U.S. hospitals were circumcised.

Today we know that the operation is not painless. We also know that it doesn't cure or prevent blindness, epilepsy, or insanity. Some of the other claims made for circumcision have also proven false. When parents and doctors began to speak out against it, circumcision became a topic of debate. Today the debate is pretty much over in most parts of the world. In Europe, for example, only two out of every hundred baby boys are circumcised. Most of these circumcisions are done for religious reasons, but, even some Jewish and Muslim parents are deciding against the operation.

In this country, the debate continues. Those in favor of circumcision argue that it helps protect against cancer of the penis, urinary tract infections in infants, and STDs. (STDs are sexually transmitted diseases—infections that can be passed through sexual contact.) Those against circumcision dispute these claims. Both sides point to studies to support their point of view.

(If you're interested in learning more about the debate, see the Resource Section at the back of this book under the heading "Circumcision" page 225.)

In the past, nearly all male babies born in this country were circumcised. Over the years, things have changed. Today only about 60 percent of babies are circumcised in the United States. More boys than ever are reaching puberty with their foreskins still intact. Nowadays, we get a lot of the questions about the foreskin and the uncircumcised penis. Circumcision doesn't have any effect on how a boy develops during puberty, though. Puberty is the same whether you've been circumcised or not. But the operation does affect the appearance of the penis.

In the next few pages, we'll give you a quickie course in the anatomy of the foreskin. We'll also explain how circumcision affects the appearance of the penis. As you'll learn, there are several different methods for doing a circumcision. Some methods leave more of the foreskin than others. The scars they leave may also differ in appearance.

The Uncircumcised Penis

In uncircumcised adult males, the foreskin can be retracted. This means it can be pulled back over the glans and slid down the shaft of the penis. The foreskin can be retracted when the penis is erect or soft. The foreskin may also retract on its own during an erection.

In most newborn babies, the foreskin cannot be retracted. In fact, it's still attached to the glans in most cases. When the baby is developing in the womb, the foreskin and glans are joined to one another by connecting tissue. The glans and foreskin will remain joined until the cells of the connecting tissue begin to shed. This process may start before birth, but it usually takes years to complete.

While the process is occurring both the glans and the foreskin are constantly shedding cells from their surfaces. These cells are shed in little nests or clumps. This creates little pockets of space between the foreskin and glans. The shed cells form little "pearls"—rounded, white or slightly yellow—lumps under the foreskin. The pearls roll around between the two surfaces until they work their way out from under the opening at the top of the foreskin.

As more cells are shed, more pockets of space are created between the foreskin and glans. Sooner or later, there is more space than there is connecting tissue. Only a few thin bands here and there still connect the glans and foreskin. Finally, these, too, dissolve. At last, the glans and foreskin are completely separated.

The foreskin can't be retracted all the way until it is completely separated from the glans. Even once the separation has occurred, the foreskin opening may be too narrow for it to be pulled back over the glans. Usually, however, the foreskin is stretched by erections, and by the actions of the boy himself. As a result, it can often be fully retracted soon after it has separated from the glans.

The stretching of the foreskin begins at an early age, because even as little babies, boys have erections from time to time. The stretching is also helped by the fact that little boys "discover" their genitals at a young age. Uncircumcised boys soon discover how good it feels to slide the foreskin back and forth across the glans. As they do this, they gradually stretch the foreskin opening.

Stages of Foreskin Retraction in Uncircumcised Males

As we've said, the foreskin doesn't become fully retractable overnight. The glans and foreskin must first separate. Even after that has occurred the foreskin opening must also be loose enough to be pulled back over the glans. The whole process usually takes many years. The timing differs from one boy to the next. It tends to happen slowly, though, a little bit at a time. Figure 18 shows five different stages in the process. If you are not

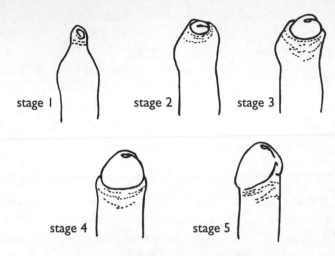

Figure 18. Five Stages of Foreskin Retraction

circumcised, Figure 18 and the descriptions below will help you decide which stage you are in now. Some boys do not go through all five stages.

- **Stage 1:** The foreskin doesn't retract at all. The foreskin opening is small and tight. This is the most common stage among newborn babies. Even boys twelve or older can be in this stage. However, only a few boys over the age of twelve are still in Stage 1.
- **Stage 2:** In this stage, you can retract the foreskin enough to see the urinary opening. This stage is most common during the first two years of life. In some cases this stage can last until a boy is twelve or over. But, less than one out of ten boys over the age of twelve are still in Stage 2.
- **Stage 3:** In this stage, the foreskin can be pulled further back. It can be retracted about halfway to the

corona, the ridge around the bottom of the glans. This is the most common stage throughout early childhood. Many boys of puberty age are still in this stage.

• **Stage 4:** The foreskin can be pulled back even further. It can retract to just above the corona, but can't be pulled over the corona itself. This stage is very common in boys between the ages of eight and eleven. But it can also be seen in babies less than a year old, and in boys over the age of sixteen.

• **Stage 5:** The foreskin can be fully retracted back over the glans, enabling the entire glans to be seen. The majority of boys between the ages of eleven and fifteen are in Stage 5. Some boys reach it as early as one or as late as eighteen. There have even been cases of newborn babies whose foreskins could be fully retracted.

There are some males whose foreskins never get to Stage 5. Experts disagree about how to deal with this. Some feel the foreskin should be left alone as long as it isn't causing pain or other problems. Others say the foreskin should be treated so it can fully retract. This can usually be done without circumcision. (See the box on page 61.)

If your foreskin isn't fully retractable, don't worry. But, if it causes pain or discomfort, see your doctor. Often, the problem can be treated with a prescription cream applied to the foreskin for a couple of weeks. If you're not having pain, it's fine to try stretching the foreskin opening yourself. You can start by gently pulling the foreskin back. Be gentle, though. Stretch slowly, over time. In the bath, when you've been soaking in warm water, is a good time for stretching. Don't stretch to the point of pain. You may be tearing tissue.

The foreskin should never be forced to retract! Forcing retraction can leave raw, bleeding areas on the glans and foreskin. As these areas heal, "skin bridges," or adhesions, may form. These are bands of tissue between the foreskin and glans that can prevent retraction. Removing them may require a doctor's care.

Also, if you force a tight foreskin to retract, it may get stuck behind the glans. If this happens, there's no need to panic. Hold the glans between your thumb and fingers and apply firm pressure for a couple of minutes. This will make it shrink enough so that the foreskin can be brought forward over the glans again. A lubricant, such as KY jelly, may also be helpful.

HANGING ONTO YOUR FORESKIN

Basic, everyday knowledge about the foreskin and its care used to be handed down from father to son. With so many men being circumcised in this country, much of the knowledge was lost.

The foreskin pretty much disappeared from medical textbooks. Most doctors knew little about the foreskin except how to remove it.

Today there is more knowledge about the foreskin. But, even now, many doctors in this country know little about its care. Problems with the foreskin are not common, but they do happen. Many doctors are quick to recommend circumcision for even the most minor problem. Many times, though, these problems can be treated in other, less drastic ways. If you develop a problem and your doctor recommends circumcision, get another opinion from a "foreskin-friendly" doctor. Ask your parents or guardian to help you find a doctor who knows about foreskins. See the resource pages at the back of this book under the heading "Circumcision" for more information.

The Anatomy of the Foreskin

The foreskin is two layers thick. The two layers can glide back and forth over each other. The top, or outer, layer is called the outer foreskin. The inner layer is called the inner foreskin. In Figure 17, you can see the outer foreskin, but not the inner foreskin. You have to retract the foreskin, or pull it away from the glans, to see the inner layer.

The outer foreskin is really just a continuation of the same skin that covers the shaft of the penis. Near the tip of the glans, the foreskin folds over on itself. At the fold, there's a band of elastic tissue called the *ridged* band. (See Figure 19.)

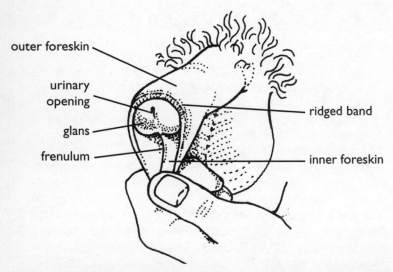

Figure 19. The Foreskin and Ridged Band. In this front-on view of a soft penis, the foreskin is pulled down to show the inner foreskin and other structures that are normally hidden.

ridged (RIJD)

The ridged band joins the outer foreskin to the inner foreskin. It is usually pinker, redder, or deeper in color than the rest of the foreskin.

The ridged band is very elastic. It works like a rubber band. During retraction, the band stretches enough to slip back over the glans and the shaft. When the foreskin is pulled forward, the band contracts and the foreskin opening returns to its normal size.

The band is a series of wrinkles, or ridges. Along these ridges are special nerve endings. These nerve endings respond to pressure. They are stimulated when the foreskin moves back and forth over the glans.

The inner foreskin isn't really skin at all. It is a special kind of tissue found nowhere else in the body. It is pink or red or deep in color, moist to the touch, and very sensitive. It, too, has many special nerve endings. Like the ridged band, it is a source of sexual pleasure for uncircumcised males. The inner foreskin is attached to the penis beneath the corona of the glans.

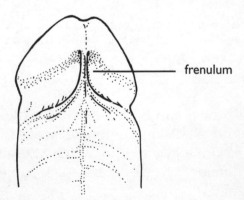

frenulum

Figure 20. The Frenulum. In this underside view of the penis, the foreskin is retracted to show the "Y" shaped frenulum. In this view the "Y" of the frenulum is shown upside down.

On the underside of the glans, there is a Y-shaped web of tissue called the *frenulum*. (See Figure 20.) Like the glans and the inner foreskin, the frenulum has many nerve endings. It is a very sensitive part of the penis. It is usually removed during circumcision, though part of it may remain.

When the outer foreskin is retracted, the inner foreskin comes into view. You can see how this works in Figure 21. The outer foreskin is pulled back over the glans. This pulls the ridged band out onto the glans. As the ridged band comes into view and moves down the shaft, the inner foreskin unrolls on the glans.

When the foreskin is fully retracted, the ridged band is about halfway down the shaft. The glans is uncovered, and you can see all of the corona.

The Circumcised Penis

> I have this band of skin on my penis. It's like a ring around my penis about halfway down. It's looks weird. How come I have this?
>
> *Anonymous, from question box*

> I have extra skin on my penis. It kinda wrinkles and bunches up behind the head [glans]. There's a brown line that goes all the way round it. Is this normal? I've always had it, as long as I can remember.
>
> *Anonymous, from question box*

These boys are both describing their circumcision scars. The extra skin one boy describes is what's left of his foreskin. As we've said, different types of operations leave different types of scars. Also, people's bodies heal differently.

frenulum (FREN-you-lum)

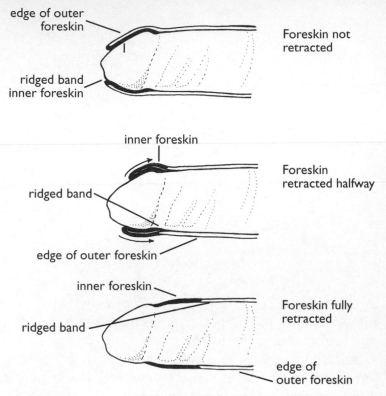

Figure 21. Retraction of the Foreskin. Notice how the foreskin has two layers and unrolls when it's retracted.

The scar is often easier to see when the penis is erect. It is also easier to see in some males than in others. But, in most circumcised males, there is a visible scar circling the shaft of the penis. In some cases, the scar is on the upper part of the shaft, near the glans. In other cases, it is further down on the shaft. Figure 22 shows the circumcision scar on a soft penis.

The texture and the color of the skin may be different in the area of the scar than on the rest of the penis. The differently colored skin is what remains of the inner

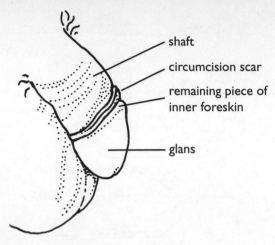

shaft

circumcision scar

remaining piece of
inner foreskin

glans

Figure 22. Circumcision Scar

foreskin. Some boys have loose skin bunched up behind the glans. This, too, is perfectly normal. Again, it is simply the remains of the foreskin.

Some circumcision operations leave part of the frenulum. What's left of this Y-shaped piece of tissue may be visible on the underside of the penis.

The glans of an circumcised penis looks a bit different from the glans of an uncircumcised penis. In uncircumcised males, the foreskin protects the glans. The glans is soft, shiny, and moist. It's like the tissue on the inside of your cheek, mouth, or on the underside of your eyelid. In circumcised boys, without the protection of the foreskin, the glans becomes covered with layers of thick, dry, hard cells. The tissue is no longer moist and shiny.

OTHER VARIATIONS IN THE PENIS

Aside from whether or not they've been circumcised, penises also differ in other ways (see Figure 23). They may be thin or fat, short or long. Veins may be visible on

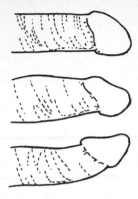

Figure 23. Different Penis Shapes. Penises come in lots of different shapes, some of which are pictured here.

the surface of the penis. The head (glans) may look wider or narrower than the shaft. The shape of the glans varies too. All these variations are normal.

The penis may hang straight down, to the left, or to the right. When it's erect, the penis may be straight, or it may curve to the left or right. It may also curve up toward the body or down toward the floor. The angle at which it sticks out from the body also varies. These variations in the erect penis are more fully described in Chapter 6.

Boys sometimes ask about *pearly penile papules* and about *lymphoceles*. They don't, of course, ask about them by name. But, that's what they're asking about when they describe the following conditions:

• **Pearly penile papules:** Some men have tiny pink bumps arranged in rows around the corona or scattered over the glans. The "pearly" in their name comes from

papules (PAP-yules)
lymphoceles (limf-oh seals)

CARE OF YOUR SEX ORGANS

All boys—circumcised or not—should wash their genitals every day. Uncircumcised boys should pull the foreskin back all the way or as far as it will comfortably go. If it can't be retracted at all, don't worry. The "pearls" between the foreskin and glans will do the cleaning for you. Just wash the outer foreskin.

If the foreskin is fully retractable, clean the glans, the inner foreskin, and all around the groove just beneath the corona. The foreskin produces *smegma*, a natural lubricant to help the foreskin slide back and forth smoothly. If it builds up under the foreskin, it causes an unpleasant odor. So rinse off any smegma you see.

Soap can sting and irritate the glans and inner foreskin. Some experts advise avoiding soap. Rinsing well with water should do the trick. If you do use soap, make sure it is very mild.

their sheen. They are more common in younger men and may disappear with age. They are completely normal. They do not cause symptoms and do not need medical treatment.

• **Lymphocele:** Sometimes the lymph glands near the corona get blocked and swell up. This can happen after injury or a lot of sexual activity. Often, though, it happens without an obvious cause. When it does, translucent, firm, worm-like swellings appear on the penis. They go away on their own within a few weeks and do not require medical treatment.

smegma (SMEG-muh)

THE SCROTUM

The scrotum may hang lower or higher than the tip of the penis. It may have some pubic hair or none. In grown men, the left side of the scrotum usually hangs lower than the right. The testicle on the right side of the scrotum is usually slightly larger than the left one.

The Raphe

> I have this line that divides my testicles and it goes all the way up the back of my penis. It looks like a scar. Do other guys have this?
>
> *Anonymous, from the question box*

This boy is asking about the *raphe.* It runs down the center of the underside of the penis. It continues along the center of the scrotum and all the way to the anus. It may be red or dark in color. It's called the raphe, and it's perfectly normal.

All males have one. It's easier to see in some than in others. Boys think the raphe has something to do with circumcision. It doesn't. The raphe is just a joining line, or seam, that was formed way back when you were developing inside your mother's womb.

"Empty" Scrotum: Absent, Undescended, and Retractile Testicles

The scrotum can be empty on one or both sides because one or both testicles are missing. A number of different medical conditions can cause an "empty" scrotum. In rare cases, a boy is born with only one testicle. Also, injury or disease can damage a testicle so badly that it

raphe (RAY-fee)

must be removed. If one testicle is missing but the other testicle is healthy, the boy will develop normally. His sex life will not be affected. The remaining testicle will produce enough sperm and he'll be able to father a child.

Undescended and *retractile* testicles are two other conditions that can cause an "empty" scrotum. The testicles develop inside the abdomen. Normally, they descend (come down) into the scrotum before birth. But sometimes one (or both) of them remain in the body. In most cases, the undescended testicles move down into the scrotum in the first six months to twelve months of the baby's life. If they don't, the baby should have an operation to bring the testicle down into the scrotum.

If it's not brought down into the scrotum, the testicle may develop cancer. In the past, doctors often waited until the boy was older to operate. But now we know that the testicle may not develop properly if it stays up in the body for too long. Therefore, doctors perform the operation while the boy is still a baby or toddler.

Before surgery the doctor will check to make sure the undescended testicle isn't really a retractile testicle. In this condition, one (or, more often, both) of the testicles pulls up to the top of the scrotum or even up into the body from time to time. Cold weather, a cold bath, excitement, or extreme physical activity can all cause the testicle to retract up into the body for a while. Then, the testicle returns to its normal position.

Since this condition usually takes care of itself by the time a boy reaches puberty, treatment usually isn't nec-

undescended (un-duh-SEN-did)
retractile (ree-TRACK-tile)

essary. But a boy with this condition needs to see a doctor regularly for checkups. In some cases, a retractile testicle fails to come back down and the doctor can't draw it back into the scrotum. Or, the testicle remains retracted most of the time. In these cases, an operation is done so the testicle stays in place.

We hope this chapter has answered your questions about your sex organs. In the next chapter, we will talk about the puberty growth spurt.

CHAPTER 4

The Puberty
Growth Spurt

Are the shoes you bought just last month too small?
Are your practically brand-new jeans up around your
ankles already? If so, you've probably started your puberty growth spurt.

During puberty, we go through a period of extra-fast
growth. We put on weight and grow taller at a faster rate
than before puberty. We call this period of super-fast
growth "the puberty growth spurt." It begins at different
ages for different boys. It is more dramatic in some boys
than in others. But all boys do a good deal of growing at
this time. This growth spurt usually lasts for a few years.
Then, the rate of growth slows back down again and
eventually stops.

In this chapter, we'll be talking about several different
aspects of the puberty growth spurt. Two of these are
the height spurt and the weight spurt. But the puberty
growth spurt does more than make you taller and heavier. It also makes you stronger. In part, this is because
your muscles get bigger. But, as you'll learn in this
chapter, this isn't the only reason you grow stronger
during puberty.

As you mature and grow, certain parts of your body grow more than others. As a result, your face and body look quite different than they did before puberty. You start to look more adult and less like a kid!

While you are growing and developing in so many different ways, eating properly and exercising are especially important, but many young people don't do either. Their diets don't have the vitamins and minerals they need and they don't get enough exercise. These problems can have a particularly bad effect on a young person's bones. During puberty you build up the bone strength that will last your whole lifetime. If you don't build enough bone mass in these years, it can cause problems later in life. Proper diet and exercise are the keys to building strong bones. However, the wrong kind of exercise can be dangerous. For example, weight lifting could possibly damage growing bones. In this chapter, you'll learn about proper diet and safe exercise during your puberty years.

THE HEIGHT SPURT

Before he hits puberty, the average boy is growing at a rate of about two inches per year. Once the height spurt begins, growth speeds up. A boy's rate of growth may nearly double, so he adds almost four inches to his height in a single year. On the average, a boy adds a total of about nine to eleven inches to his height during the puberty growth spurt.

The growth spurt usually lasts about three or four years. Then the rate of growth slows down again. This does not mean that a boy stops growing altogether. Most boys continue to grow taller until they get to about the age of nineteen. Some even continue to grow in their twenties. But the period of extra-fast growth lasts only a few years.

Girls go through a height spurt during puberty, too. But girls typically start their height spurts earlier than boys. For girls, the growth spurt happens early in puberty. It is one of the first changes. For boys, the growth spurt is not an early change. It happens later in puberty.

On average, boys' growth spurts happen about two years later than girls' growth spurts. This is why eleven- and twelve-year-old boys are often shorter than the girls their age. But, a couple of years later, the boys start their growth spurt. Then, the boys usually catch up to the girls and eventually pass them in height. Often an eleven- or twelve-year-old boy who is shorter than the girls his age will be taller than they are by thirteen or fourteen.

How Tall Will I Be?

We can't tell for sure how tall you'll be. But we can give you a couple of clues.

Your height *before* your growth spurt is one clue. If you are short as a child, it's likely you'll be short as an adult. Likewise, tall children tend to become tall adults. But this is *definitely* not a hard and fast rule. We spoke with many men who were among the shortest in their class before puberty, but among the tallest after puberty.

You can get a better idea of your adult height by following the steps below. First, though, you need to know how tall your mom and dad are. (For this exercise, guardians, foster, and adoptive parents won't do. You need to know your birth parents' heights.)

1. Add 5 inches to your dad's height.
2. Add your mom's height to the result you got in Step #1.
3. Take the result you got in Step #2 and divide it by 2 to get your estimated adult height.

Example: Greg's father is 5 feet, 10 inches tall, and his mother is 5 feet, 7 inches tall.

1. First we add 5 inches to his father's height. The result is 5 feet, 15 inches.

2. Now add his mother's height (5 feet, 7 inches) to the result we got in Step #1 (5 feet, 15 inches). The result is 10 feet, 22 inches.

3. Now we divide the result from Step # 2 (10 feet, 22 inches) by 2. The result is 5 feet, 11 inches. This is Greg's estimated adult height.

Probably your parents are not the same height as Greg's parents. You will have to do the math for yourself, using your parents' heights. Remember, though, the result is only an estimate. Your actual adult height may be more or less than this.

Tall Tales and Short Stories

The tallest man who ever lived was eight feet, eleven inches tall. The shortest was only 2 feet, 2 ½ inches. But these were very unusual cases. Most men (9 out of 10) will be between five feet, six inches, and six feet, two inches, tall. The average height for grown men is five feet, ten inches tall.

We asked men, "What's the one thing you would most like to change about your body?"

"My height" was second only to penis size in their answers. No one wished to be shorter. Nearly all wished to be taller. Even men a couple of inches taller than average, said they "wouldn't mind" being a bit taller. One shorter-than-average man had this to say:

> I'm only five feet, six inches. Being short has always bugged me. People make cracks, call you "shrimp" or "shortie." I'm really coordinated and good at sports. Being short made it difficult to get on the team in high school. I guess I compensated

by getting into weight lifting and concentrating on wrestling. In a way, though, now that I'm older, it turns out that being short was kind of an advantage. It made me really concentrate on working out and developing a strong, muscular body—a habit that's stayed with me. I still work out. I'm in great physical shape, whereas a lot of guys my age are overweight and flabby and out of shape. I'm healthier than a lot of guys. Maybe if I'd been taller I wouldn't have gotten so into working out and taking care of my body. Still, to tell the truth, I wish I were taller.

Harold, age 34

Very tall men aren't always happy about their height:

I'm six foot seven. I'm always looking down on other people. People are always saying dumb things like, "How is the weather up there?" I was this tall when I was fourteen. I always felt like a freak. I kind of slouched and hunched over, trying not to look so tall. My mother was always yelling at me to stand up straight. I still have terrible posture. I'm in my forties now, so it's not so bad anymore. There are little inconveniences, like bumping your head and trying to scrunch into cars. But, it's not like when I was a teenager. It really bothered me then. Being different was difficult.

Frank, age 43

Some men have a very positive attitude. It doesn't matter if they are shorter than average:

I've always been short, even as a kid. So I've had a whole lifetime to adjust. It's really not a problem for me like it is for some guys. I know lots of short guys who are always kind of cocky, on the defensive, who talk loud or always act the clown or are kind of brash or pushy. They're sort of making up for the fact that they're short, acting big so that people will notice them. Like they might get missed or passed over because they're short. But I don't really feel that need. I'm short and I'm a pretty quiet guy. But I still feel that people take note of me because I'm comfortable with myself, the way I am. I think people notice or feel that kind of satisfaction when you're at peace with yourself and accept yourself the way you are.

Rick, age 39

Rick went on to explain that being short can cause dating problems.

There's a sort of unwritten rule that the guy has to be taller than the girl. All the girls were always taller than me. So I realized early on that I wasn't going to pay attention to that rule. Because if I only asked out girls who were shorter than me . . . well, I wouldn't have gone out on too many dates. So I just ignored that rule and asked out whomever I wanted.

I got turned down sometimes, just on account of my height. There were girls, and later women, who even though they'd go out with me were bothered by my being short. They'd wear flat-heeled shoes instead of the high heels they probably would have worn. But once I got involved with someone, you know, seriously, we'd kid around and it was never a real problem.

It's true that a lot of people follow this rule about the guy having to be taller. It does affect you. Maybe it's a little harder to get a date, to find a girl who isn't uptight about it. My wife, by the way, is five inches taller than me and wears high heels. It doesn't bother her that there's a difference in our height. It is breaking that unwritten law, though, and people do look at us. I figure that's their problem.

Rick, age 39

Rick has a healthy attitude about himself. He doesn't seem to worry about what other people think. But there's no getting around it. Our society puts a lot of importance on a man's height. In fact, many people are prejudiced against short men. You're probably familiar with racial prejudice. People who have racial prejudices discriminate against others with a different skin color. Prejudice against short men isn't as obvious as racial prejudice, but, it does exist. For example, two men might apply for a job. Studies show that a tall man is more likely than a short man to get the job, simply because he's tall.

Since many (but not all) people have these prejudices, it's not surprising that short men often wish they were taller. The fact is, you can't do much about your height. You *can* do something about the way you deal with it. You can go out there and be all the other things you want to be. You don't have to be six feet tall to be a good

---

PILLS THAT MAKE YOU TALLER???

No, there's no magic pill to make you taller. But scientists are now able to make growth *hormone* in an injectable form as a shot. Growth hormone is a chemical made by the body. It helps to control our growth and development.

Doctors use growth hormone to treat certain medical problems. For example, it is used to treat kids whose bodies don't make enough growth hormone. These boys and girls are unusually short as children. Their problem is treated long before puberty. Growth hormone is also used to treat kids with other illnesses that affect their height.

In the past, some doctors prescribed growth hormone to perfectly healthy kids who just happened to be short. This is no longer recommended. Growth hormone can speed up a kid's growth for a year or two. But it probably doesn't make them any taller as adults. Besides, growth hormone can cause side effects like liver damage. That's why most doctors feel growth hormone should not be used unless there's a lack of the naturally produced hormone or specific illnesses affecting growth.

---

hormone (HOR-moan)

friend. There are no height requirements when it comes to being funny, or smart, or a good athlete. You may not be able to change your height, but you can still achieve your goals!

Think of the many shorter-than-average men who have become famous stars. There are actors like Michael J. Fox and Tom Cruise, and baseball immortals like Phil Rizzuto and Ty Cobb, among many others. Knowing this in your head is one thing. When you really believe it with your heart, you will feel okay about yourself no matter how short or tall you are.

Feet First

You get taller because the height spurt makes the bones in the trunk of your body and legs grow longer. Some bones start the growth spurt before others, though. The bones in your feet and hands start to grow before other bones. Your feet reach their adult size before you've reached your adult height. Next the bones in the lower arm and lower leg start their growth spurt. They are followed by the bones in upper arm and thigh. Your trunk is the last part of your body to reach adult size. When it does, you will be at your adult height.

THE WEIGHT SPURT

During your puberty growth spurt, you get heavier as well as taller. In fact, during puberty, boys increase their weight more than at any other time in their lives. We call this period of extra-fast weight gain "the weight spurt." Part of it is due to the growth of bones and internal organs. Part of it is also due to the bigger muscles boys grow at this time.

Like the height spurt, the weight spurt lasts three to four years. Then, the rate at which you gain weight

GROWING PAINS AND SCOLIOSIS

Growing pains can be a real pain! They're not serious, but they're not much fun either. They are most common in thirteen year olds, but younger and older boys also have them.

The pains are not constant. They come and go. They cause a dull, painful, achy feeling. They're often felt behind the knee, in the thigh, or along the shin. They may also occur in the arms, back, groin, shoulders, or ankles. Doctors don't really know what causes growing pains.

Growing pains usually don't need medical treatment. They eventually go away on their own. Until they do, massages, a heating pad, and a nonaspirin pain reliever should help. If the pain is severe or doesn't go away, check it out with a doctor— just to make sure the pain isn't due to something more serious.

Scoliosis is another "growing" problem. It's an abnormal curve in the spine. It's not like the slumped-forward kind of curve from poor posture. Rather, the curve is to the left or right. It may result in one hip or shoulder being higher than the other. Or, the curve may have an "S" shape. Sometimes, one shoulder blade stands out, or the body has a kind of list. Scoliosis tends to run in families, but, in most cases, the cause is not known.

Many cases are very mild and don't require more than some simple exercises. Even if the exercises can't correct the actual curvature, they can help get rid of the pain that can result from the body being thrown out of balance by the curvature. In some cases, treatment may require wearing a back brace for a time. Today these braces are light and less bulky than in the past. They can be worn under clothing so they don't show. More serious cases may require surgery.

Scoliosis is easiest to correct if it is treated early. It's best to start checking for the first signs before puberty begins. In some grade schools, this is done by a school doctor. If it's not done at your school, ask your doctor to check your spine.

scoliosis (skoh-lee-OH-sis)

slows back down. During the weight spurt, a boy may gain twenty pounds in a single year. Over the course of the entire weight spurt, the average weight gain is forty-five to fifty pounds. Of course, we're not all average, and you may gain more or less than this. Most boys, though, will add between forty to sixty pounds during their weight spurt.

Your Changing Shape

If growing up were simply a matter of getting bigger, adults would look like giant babies. (We may *act* like big babies at times, but adults don't *look* like big babies.) But, some parts of our bodies grow more than others, so that our body *proportions* change. In other words, there's a change in the size of certain parts in relation to other parts.

The drawing of the adult man and the baby in Figure 24 shows them both at the same height. This makes it easier to see how body proportions change. For example, the baby's head is large compared to other parts of his body. It accounts for one-fourth of his total size. But the man's head only accounts for one-eighth of his height.

Look, too, at how wide the head is compared to the shoulders. On the baby, the head is nearly as wide as the shoulders. On the man, the head is nowhere near as broad as his shoulders. Also, the man's legs account for nearly half his height. The baby's legs are a much smaller part of his total size.

Puberty causes dramatic changes in our body proportions. Your legs grow quite a bit during the puberty growth spurt. And since your shoulders get broader,

proportions (pruh-POR-shuns)

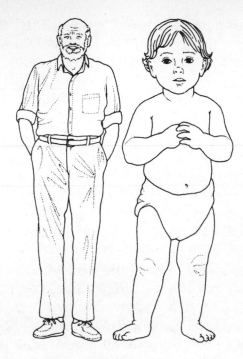

Figure 24. Adult Male and Giant Baby

your hips seem narrower in comparison. Your shoulders also become more muscular. In fact, the muscles all over your body grow larger, especially in your thighs, calves, and upper arms. Your whole body begins to look less like a boy's body and more like a man's.

Even the proportions of your face change. The lower part of your face lengthens. Your chin juts out more. Your hairline moves further back and your forehead widens. As a result, your face is longer, narrower, and less pudgy than when you were a kid. Your face, too, looks more adult.

Because you see yourself in the mirror each day, these changes may not be real obvious to you, but look at class pictures over a few years and you'll see the change. Of course, face changes are more dramatic in some boys than in others.

THE STRENGTH SPURT

A boy's strength increases during puberty. It's during this time that boys become stronger than girls. Typically, a boy of sixteen is twice as strong as he was at twelve.

Some of this increase in strength comes from an increase in the size of your muscles. Your muscles grow bigger during the puberty weight spurt. In fact, muscle tissue accounts for much of the weight boys gain during puberty.

However, muscle size alone isn't enough to explain the increase in a boy's strength. The strength spurt is due, in large part, to *testosterone.*

Testosterone is a hormone made in the testicles. During puberty a boy begins making increasing amounts of this hormone. Testosterone causes growth of the penis, facial hair, pubic hair, other body hair, and many other puberty changes. In fact, it's what causes the increase in muscle tissue in the first place.

Testosterone also causes changes in muscle fibers. It alters the way muscles work, increasing their strength. Testosterone doesn't just make muscles bigger. It also makes them work better!

The increase in strength doesn't happen right away. First, the muscles increase in size. Then, the increase in strength follows some months later.

Typically, the strength spurt comes later in puberty. It comes after the period of fastest growth and weight. The

testosterone (tes-TOS-tuh-roan)

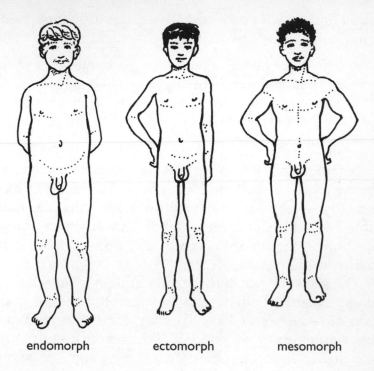

endomorph   ectomorph   mesomorph

Figure 25. Three Body Types

sex organs are usually fairly well developed by then. The increase in strength continues beyond puberty and into the early twenties.

Basic Body Types

Not all boys of the same weight are equally strong. Some boys may be stronger because they are more fit or exercise more often. But, no matter how much they exercise, some boys will never be as strong as others. The difference has to do with basic body types.

Some boys think they're not muscular enough. Or, they think they're overweight when they're not. They don't understand about body types. There are three basic body types (See Figure 25).

- *Endomorphs* tend to have rounder bodies with more body fat and softer curves.
- *Ectomorphs* are slim, less curvy, and more angular.
- *Mesomorphs* are muscular, with wide shoulders and relatively slim hips.

If you're an endomorph, it's important for you to know that your body is meant to be rounder. You may be in good physical shape, yet look less muscular than your friends or classmates who are mesomorphs. Pound for pound, mesomorphs have more muscle tissue than endomorphs or ectomorphs.

The hunk models in magazines and on TV may have a more muscular body type than yours. If that's the case, you can never really look like they do. It doesn't matter how much exercise you do. Before you jump to the conclusion that you're not muscular enough, take your basic body type into account.

To some extent, you can change the shape of your body by diet and exercise. If you're thin, you can put on weight. If you're fat, you can diet and exercise so that your body loses some of its fat tissue. Once you're making enough testosterone, you can build up your muscles by working out with weights. (But, read the next section, "Weight Training," before you run off to bench press 250 lbs.) Remember, though, you do have a basic body shape that can't be changed no matter what type of exercise you do.

endomorphs (EN-doe-morfs)
ectomorphs (ECK-toe-morfs)
mesomorphs (MEZ-oh-morfs)

STEROIDS

Steroids are a class of hormones made by the body. Testosterone is one example of a steroid hormone. In the 1950s, man-made steroids were developed for use in treating cancer and other serious diseases.

Some boys, and men, too, take these drugs to make their bodies build bulging muscles. But steroids are dangerous, especially during puberty. They can stunt your body's normal growth. They can also make your testicles shrink and your breasts enlarge. And they also cause moodiness, violent behavior (known as "roid rage"), and other mental problems. In the long run, steroids may increase a person's risk of heart attack and liver cancer.

Steroids can be habit-forming, making it hard for a person to stop their use. Because of all these medical problems, athletes in major competitions, like the Olympics, are tested for steroid use and disqualified if tests show they've used these drugs. Steroids just aren't a good idea. If you really want to build muscles, you can get good results safely with proper exercise.

Weight Training

Weight training means working out on body-building machines and lifting weights. This type of exercise is also called strength training. Like any form of exercise, it has all sorts of benefits. (Far too many of us are total couch potatoes!) If you're thinking about getting into weight training, our advice is, "Go for it!"

But (you knew there was going to be a but, didn't you?) don't expect to build up bulging muscles until you reach the later stages of puberty. You simply can't

steroids (STAIR-oyds)

build big muscles until your body is making enough testosterone.

Also, be sure you go about weight training in the right way. Otherwise, you could do serious damage to your body and even stunt your growth. Here's why: During your growth spurt, the long bones in your arms and legs do a lot of growing. Growth happens at the ends of these long bones. The growing part of the bone is soft and subject to injury. Accidents or other injuries can break this soft part or separate it from the rest of the bone. The result may be stunted or uneven growth. The injured arm or leg might, for example, wind up being shorter than its mate.

During the height spurt your bones are growing at their fastest rate. Injuries can also happen at the point where the muscle attaches to the growing part of the bone. This is less serious than separations and breaks, but, it often requires medical treatment.

Because of the risks, weight training should only be done in a carefully supervised program. (Never do weight lifting alone.) Before you start any exercise program, talk to your doctor about the type and intensity of exercise that is safe for you, at your stage of development. Then, work with your coach or instructor on a specific training program. Always stay within the guidelines set by your doctor and coach.

TAKING CARE OF YOUR BODY

Eating Right and Exercising

To grow, your body needs enough of many different nutrients. To get all the nutrients you need, you must eat a variety of foods. Figure 26 shows what types of food and how many servings of each type you should eat each day.

Your bones grow thicker and stronger during puberty. To grow properly, they need plenty of minerals, such as *calcium* and *zinc*. Your body also needs vitamins, like vitamin D, to carry the calcium to your bones. Not getting enough of these minerals and vitamins can stunt your growth and permanently weaken your bones.

In fact, when it comes to bones, puberty is just about the most important time in your life. During puberty, you build the bone structure that will support you for all the rest of your years. As you get older, as part of the natural process of aging, your bones become weaker. During puberty you are making "deposits" in your "bone bank." Later in life, you'll need to draw on the deposits you made when you were young. If you haven't built strong bones during puberty, you could run into trouble later on.

Studies show that boys are likely to get only about half the calcium they need in their diets. Doctors and public health officials are concerned about the longterm effects. To avoid problems in the future, be sure you get enough calcium in your diet. Foods rich in calcium include calcium-fortified nonfat milk, calcium-fortified soy milk, yogurt, cheese, other dairy products, calcium-fortified cereals, calcium-fortified orange juice, broccoli, kale, green beans, and tofu. Teenagers should get at least 1,300 milligrams of calcium daily. An 8 ounce glass of fortified nonfat milk contains about 300 milligrams. Fortified orange juice usually provides about the same

calcium (KAL-see-um)
zinc (ZINK)

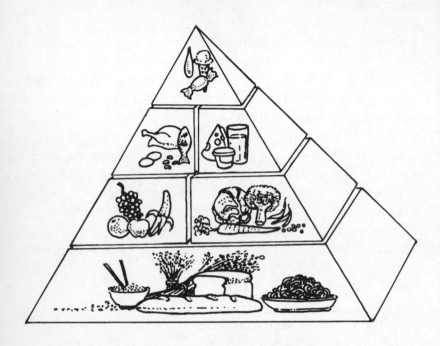

Figure 26. Food Pyramid. The Food Pyramid is a guide to help you choose a healthy diet. The box on the next page suggests the number of servings to eat from each of six food groups. Vary your diet by choosing different foods within each food group. This helps ensure a correct balance of vitamins, minerals, and other beneficial nutrients. In the different food groups, there is a range for the number of servings—like 6–11 servings from the Bread, Cereal, Rice, and Pasta group. The smaller number is for a diet of 1600 calories per day and the larger number for a diet of 2800 calories per day. An average teenager needs 2200 to 2500 calories per day, and should use the mid to upper number of servings.

WHAT COUNTS AS ONE SERVING?

Bread, Cereal, Rice, and Pasta Group
(6-11 servings)
   1 slice of bread
   1 ounce (oz) of ready-to-eat cereal
   (check labels: 1 oz = 1 to 2 cups, depending on cereal)
   1/2 cup of cooked cereal, rice, or pasta
   1/2 hamburger roll, bagel, English muffin
   3 or 4 plain crackers (small)

Vegetable Group (3-5 servings)
   1 cup of raw leafy vegetables
   1/2 cup of other vegetables, cooked or chopped raw
   3/4 cup of vegetable juice

Fruit Group (2-4 servings)
   1 medium apple, banana, orange, nectarine, peach
   1/2 cup of chopped, cooked, or canned fruit
   3/4 cup of fruit juice

Milk, Yogurt, and Cheese Group (2-3 servings)
   1 cup of milk or yogurt
   1 1/2 ounces of natural cheese
   2 ounces of process cheese

Meat, Poultry, Fish, Dry Beans, Eggs, and Nuts Group
(2-3 servings)
   2 to 3 ounces of cooked lean meat, poultry, or fish
   (1/2 cup of cooked dry beans, 1 egg or 2 tablespoons of
   peanut butter counts as 1 ounce of lean meat)

Fats, Oils, and Sweets (Use Sparingly)
   No specific serving size is given for the group because the
   message is to use sugar and oil sparingly and to avoid fatty
   meats and other fatty foods. However, some oil or fat is
   needed for good health. They supply energy and essential
   fatty acids and promote absorption of fat-soluble vitamins.

amount of calcium as fortified nonfat milk. (It's easy to know which foods are calcium-fortified, because the packages say so—usually in large type.) If you can't drink milk or don't like it, you should ask your doctor about a supplement to make sure you get that all-important calcium.

Exercise

Besides eating right, we all need regular exercise. Because your heart and lungs grow larger during puberty, your body can handle more exercise. And it *needs* it. Exercise helps you achieve your best weight. In fact, not exercising may be the most important factor that causes people to be overweight. It may be even more important than overeating, although the two tend to go together.

But exercise is more than just a tool to help you build muscles and keep your weight down. Exercise strengthens your heart, increases your energy level, sends more *oxygen* to all parts of your body.

Exercise also helps deposit calcium in the bones. This is especially important during your teens. Remember, this is when you are building up the bone mass that will sustain you for the rest of your life.

Participation in organized sports can be an excellent source of exercise. Your school may require a physical exam before joining a sports program. If it doesn't, you should see your own doctor. Most likely he'll clear you for full participation in the sport. But, if there are any restrictions on what you can do, it's good to find out before you start.

oxygen (OX-suh-gin)

As we said earlier, puberty is a time when growing bones are prone to injury. Other athletes face the same risks as boys who weight train. If any repetitive part of your sports activity (like pitching or running) causes pain, talk it over right away with your coach or doctor. You may just need a change in your training schedule. Remember, it's important to be careful with your growing body.

Tobacco, Alcohol, and Other Drugs

You can't grow a healthy body if you're using drugs, alcohol, or tobacco. You've probably already learned in school about the dangers of these substances. It's especially important to avoid using them during puberty when your body is growing. Alcohol, for example, robs the body of the calcium and zinc needed to grow strong bones.

You may feel a lot of peer pressure to use tobacco, drugs, or alcohol. In addition to peer pressure, you must also resist advertisers' efforts to get you to use alcohol or tobacco.

You probably know that tobacco is habit-forming. It can be very hard to stop smoking once you've started. You may even know that most smokers start during their teens. No wonder the giant tobacco companies have aimed so much advertising at young people. From their point of view, your teen years are very important. They are the years when they have the best chance to hook you as a long-term smoker.

Studies show that people who have a healthy lifestyle during their teen years tend to stay fit for their entire lives. Not using alcohol, tobacco, or drugs, and eating right and getting regular exercise are the main keys to that healthy lifestyle.

FEELING GOOD ABOUT YOUR BODY

A healthy body is a good body in our book. It would be nice if we could all just look at our bodies and say, "Hey, I like the way I look." But we live in a society where competition is a way of life. People compete, companies compete, even countries compete. We are always comparing and competing to see who's best. But who decides what's best?

Most of us get our ideas about what's the "best" or "most attractive" male body from the pictures we see in magazines and billboards and from television and movies. Right now, in our country, these pictures usually show tall men with big, bulging muscles. They usually have handsome, regular features, no pimples, slim waists, small rear ends, and broad chests. As you may have noticed, not too many men actually look like this.

But you wouldn't know it to look at the media. The media constantly bombard us with pictures of these tall, muscular, handsome men. They can make you feel like something about our own body is somehow not right. If you don't look like these men, you may be unhappy with the way you do look. After all, these are the men who are the heroes in the movies. They get the girls. They wind up being successful. What message does that send to those males who aren't tall, muscular, or good-looking in that particular way? With all these images of perfect "hunks," it's easy to get to thinking that these kind of bodies actually *are* better or more attractive. If you feel this way sometimes, it helps to remember that these bodies seem more desirable only because they are in fashion. And what's in fashion depends on our particular culture and our particular time. Being in fashion doesn't make one pair of jeans "better" than another.

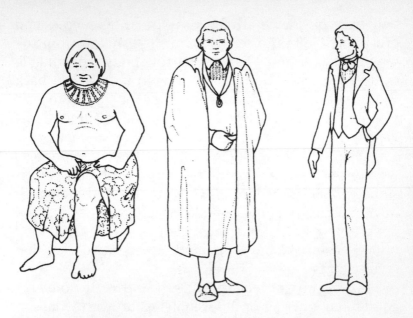

Figure 27. Fashions in Appearance. From the left are a Polynesian king, a seventeenth-century German burghermeister, and a nineteenth-century Englishman.

Being in fashion doesn't make one body type better than another, either.

It helps, too, to think about how fashions change and vary from culture to culture. The drawings you see in Figure 27 show bodies that have been in fashion in other times and other cultures. The first drawing is a Polynesian king. Most people in our society would find him grossly overweight, yet in his culture he's considered a fine figure of a man. His huge belly is taken as a sign of his masculinity. The seventeenth-century German in the second drawing would also be considered chunky by our standards. Yet, in his own day and age, his bulk was considered attractive, a sign of his success and prosperity. The third fellow is an Englishman from the nineteenth century. His thin, narrow body looks fragile compared to the "hunk" body now in fashion. Yet back then, in England, he was the type of guy who had women swooning. In fact, back then, one of our modern-day hunks might have been considered a real freak.

It also helps to remember that not everyone agrees with or goes along with the fashions of the day. For instance, there are plenty of women who find men with huge muscles popping out all over gross. Many women prefer thin men. And for most people, it's not what kind of body you have but what kind of person you are that really counts.

Learning to appreciate yourself and your body, regardless of whether or not it matches up with what's in fashion, is a big step in growing up. It's also a big step in becoming more attractive, because if you learn to like your own looks, other people will, too. It won't matter whether you have the so-called best or most attractive kind of body—not one bit. We guarantee it.

CHAPTER 5

Pimples, Perspiration, Body Hair, Shaving, and Other Changes

First off, we want to point out that this chapter isn't a complete bummer. After all, it covers shaving and the growth of facial and body hair. Most boys are at least a little jazzed about starting to shave. Growing chest hair and other body hair are also "manly" milestones. But, we have to admit that a lot of this chapter deals with the down side of puberty. Body odor and zits, cracking voices, and even swollen breasts: Yikes! These are nobody's idea of a good time. Over the years, we've seen many boys excited about starting puberty. They can't wait to develop stronger muscles and start shaving. But we've yet to come across a boy who "couldn't wait" to get his first pimple.

Zits, body odor, cracking voices, and breast changes are less-than-wonderful parts of puberty. We won't try to pretend otherwise. Instead, we'll give you the facts, so you know what to expect. We won't leave it at that though. We'll also give you some tips on how to cope. We'll tell you about *acne* treatments and ways of coping

acne (AK-nee)

with body odor. So, hang in there. The downside isn't really so terrible. And, remember, growing up also has its upside. (See the box on page 118 for an upside look at puberty.)

UNDERARM AND BODY HAIR

During puberty, hair starts to grow in places where it never grew before. You grow pubic, underarm, and facial hair. Darker hair may grow on your arms and legs as well. Hair may also start to grow on your chest and elsewhere.

Underarm hair may start growing anytime during the puberty years. Most boys grow pubic hair before hair starts to grow on their underarms. On average, boys start growing underarm hair a year or two after the first pubic hairs appear.

Hair may also start to grow on your chest. Some boys grow hair on their shoulders, backs, or buttocks. Some grow hair on the backs of their hands. Some boys become really hairy; others have very little body hair.

A Hairy Question

How hairy will you be? Boys usually take after the men in their families when it comes to body hair. If the men in your family tend to have lots of body hair, you probably will, too. If they tend to have little body hair, you probably won't have much either. Once again, this isn't a hard and fast rule. But hairiness (or lack of hair) does tend to "run in families."

Just as there are a lot of myths about penis size, there are also lots of myths about body hair. Some people believe that men with a lot of body hair are more manly than other men. This is nonsense. Body hair (or lack of body hair) doesn't have anything to do with how much of a man you are. Some people (both men *and* women) find lots of body hair attractive. Others prefer smoother, less hairy bodies. But for most people, it doesn't matter that much one way or the other. If you've worried about the amount of body hair you have, you shouldn't bother. For one thing, worrying won't make any difference. Besides, what kind of person decides whom to like on the basis of body hair?

FACIAL HAIR

As a boy goes through puberty, he also starts to grow hair on his face. His mustache, sideburns, whiskers, and beard begin to develop. The first of this facial hair doesn't usually appear until a boy's sex organs are fairly well-developed. It usually appears when he's in Stage 4 of genital development (see Figure 13 on page 37). The average boy will develop his first facial hair between the ages of fourteen and sixteen. Some boys, though, will notice this hair when they're younger. Others won't get any until they're nineteen or twenty.

Usually, the first facial hairs will appear at the outer corners of your upper lip. At first, there won't be many and they may not be very dark in color. As you get older, they will get darker and there will be more of them. Your mustache will gradually fill out, from the outer corners toward the middle of your lips. As your mustache fills out, hairs usually begin to grow on the upper part of your cheeks. Your sideburns and hair below the center of your lower lips may also grow at this time.

As you continue to mature, your facial hair will get still thicker and darker. Your beard and mustache may be the same color as the hair on your head, or they may be a different color. You may find that by age eighteen, your beard and mustache are as full and thick as they're ever going to be. However, many men keep developing facial hair into their twenties. A man may have little facial hair when he is in his teens but may have a thick beard, or a bushy mustache and sideburns by age thirty.

Shaving

Some grown men shave every day. Those who have thick, fast-growing beards, may even shave twice a day. Others grow mustaches, sideburns, or full beards. It is a personal thing, a matter of individual taste.

The men we talked to shaved their first facial hair. Some of them decided to grow a moustache or beard later in life. One man with a mustache told us:

> I don't shave it now. When I was a teenager I did, though— because it was just these few scrawny hairs. It looked pretty pathetic, kind of scraggly. It didn't look like a real mustache.
>
> *Phil, age 30*

Another man said:

> I don't shave anymore, just too lazy to shave every day. When I got that first peach fuzz, I shaved every day, religiously. It was kind of a macho thing. Also, I don't know if it's true or not, but I heard the more you shave, the faster your mustache and beard would grow in.
>
> *Ted, age 36*

A lot of the boys we talked to felt excited about shaving and looked upon shaving as a sign of growing up. Many boys wished they had as much facial hair as some of their friends had. One man told a funny story about this:

> I ran around with my cousin, Albert, and his friends, who were all in their mid-twenties. I was, say, nineteen. Albert had a car. . . . So it was really exciting for me to run around with these older guys. I wanted to look as old as them, so I'd get my

mother's eyebrow pencil and color my mustache in. You know—to make me look more mature.

So we go to a dance, and afterward I'm smooching with this gal in the back seat of Albert's car, and my mustache smears off all over her face. Jeez, talk about embarrassing. I thought I'd never live it down!

Charlie, age 67

Getting their first razor is a big event for some boys. Some bought the razor themselves. Others got theirs as gifts. Some used their dad's razor at first.

When I first started shaving, I didn't say anything to anyone. I didn't want to buy one [a razor] and just leave it there in the bathroom 'cause I knew my family would just tease me to death about it. I really didn't have that much to shave. So I just used my dad's razor.

My sisters were starting to shave their legs, and they were using dad's razor, too. He'd get hopping mad 'cause he'd go to shave his face and the blade would be dull and nicked 'cause my sisters and I used it all the time. He'd cut his face all up and then he'd start hollerin', "Who's been using my razor?" My sisters and I would say, "Not me, not me!" Finally he went out and bought us all razors and told us, "You kids use my razor again and I'll kill you."

Sam, age 35

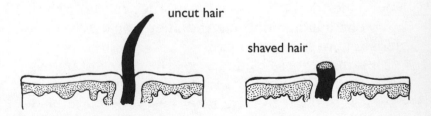

uncut hair

shaved hair

Figure 28. Hair Looks Thicker. Before shaving, the uncut hair comes to a thin tip. After shaving, the hair is cut in its thickest part making the cut hair look thicker.

DOES IT REALLY GROW BACK THICKER AND DARKER?

No, shaving doesn't really make hair grow back thicker and darker. It may look that way, though.

Hairs taper to a point at the end. The hair shaft is thinner at the tip than in the middle or at the root. Shaving cuts the hair in its thickest part (see Figure 28).

If you've never shaved, much of what's visible above the skin's surface is the thin, tapered part of each shaft. Once you shave, the thin, tapered tips are gone. All you see is the thickest part of each hair shaft.

Your hair isn't really any thicker. Sure looks that way, though.

Razors and Shavers: A Buyer's Guide

You have a choice of blade razors or electric shavers. Some men prefer the convenience of electrics. The cordless electrics are especially popular. There are two types of electric razors: foil and rotary.

Electric shavers don't require shaving cream. You don't have to change blades. They are easy to carry around. You're also less likely to cut yourself with an electric. But, a good electric shaver isn't cheap. They run from thirty up to one hundred dollars. And, they won't give you as close a shave as a blade razor.

Most men choose blade razors. The two most popular types are the disposable and the cartridge razors. With one, you throw the entire razor away when the blade gets dull. With the other, you discard the blade cartridge, but keep the rest of the razor for use with a new cartridge. Most men prefer the cartridge type.

You also have a choice of single- or twin- or even

triple-blade razors. You'll probably like the closer shave you get from a twin- or triple-blade razor. Many razors have pivoting heads or flexible blades. With these features you can get a closer shave and are less likely to cut yourself.

Twin-or triple-blade razors are more likely to cause ingrown hairs. If you're prone to ingrown hairs, you may want to try an electric razor. (See pages 113 to 114 for more information on ingrown hairs.)

You might talk to your dad or another man you trust to find out what he recommends.

Shaving Tips: Blade Razors

These tips should help you shave smoothly and safely with a blade razor.

- **Make sure your blades are clean, sharp, and free of nicks.** Change blades at least every four or five shaves. A dull blade will pull, or drag, on your skin. This causes a painful rash called "razor burn." Dropping a razor can cause hard-to-see nicks in the blade. If you drop it, chuck it!
- **Wet the hair first.** Give the hair a minute or so to soak up the water. Warm water expands and softens hair, making it easier to cut and reducing razor drag. Many men shave just after they shower. The hot water and steam do a good job of softening the beard. Your beard is toughest on the chin and upper lip. Shave these areas last to give the water more time to soften this tough part of your beard.
- **Use shaving cream or gel, not soap.** Creams and gels reduce the drag of the razor on your skin. They also soften the hair. Soap dulls blades and hardens hair, making shaving more difficult.

- **Go easy and rinse often.** Don't mash the razor into your skin. Use a light touch. Try not to go over and over the same area. Rinse your razor often to keep the blade free of hair.
- **Shave in the right direction.** Shaving against the direction of hair growth gives the closest shave. Shaving in the direction of hair growth is easier on the skin, though. On most of your face, you can shave downwards, with the hair growth. But, some men shave under their chins in an upward direction, against the hair growth. Never shave against the hair growth if you are prone to ingrown hairs.
- **Rinse with cool water and pat dry.** Rinsing with cool water closes pores and soothes skin. Pat, rather than rub, dry. You can use shaving lotions. Be careful of shaving lotions with alcohol. They can irritate the skin.
- **Never lend or borrow a razor.** Don't share. You risk sharing an infection.
- **Treat skin irritations promptly.** If you get a skin irritation after shaving, use 2.5 to 5 percent benzoyl peroxide.

Shaving Tips: Electric Shavers

Here are a few tips for getting the best shave from an electric.

- **Shave when your face is dry.**
- **Go easy.** Don't mash the shaver into your face. Pressing too hard won't give you a closer shave. Move the rotary type razor in a circular motion and the foil type up and down.
- **Clean the heads.** Follow the manufacturer's directions. If you use a rotary shaver, you'll probably

want to brush off the rotors every month or two. With a foil shaver, pop off the shaving foil and shake out the whiskers after every shave.

PERSPIRATION AND BODY ODOR

You run up and down the stairs ten times in a row. Or, maybe it's just a sizzling hot summer day. What happens?

You sweat, of course. When temperatures soar or you work out, your sweat glands swing into action. They pour out the sweat. Stress, fear, and other strong emotions can also trigger your sweat glands.

You have millions of sweat glands. They're in nearly every inch of skin on your body. They keep you from overheating by pouring out sweat. Sweat is 99 percent water, with a little bit of salt thrown in the mix. The water quickly evaporates, cooling you down. And the salt in the sweat helps draw more water from your body.

During puberty, the output from your sweat glands increases, and special sweat glands in your underarms and genital area become active for the first time. This means you sweat more and in more places. You may notice more sweat on your forehead, upper lip, neck, and chest when you exercise. Fear or worry, on the other hand, usually causes sweat in the armpits, palms, and soles of your feet. Even if you're fearless and worry-free, you'll probably sweat a lot in these areas. The reason: these areas have more sweat glands than other parts of the body.

Your body odor also changes during puberty. Sweat, by itself, doesn't cause an unpleasant odor. It is nearly odorless. But bacteria that live on human skin break the sweat down, and this causes an odor. These bacteria particularly like sweat from those special glands in your armpits and genital area that get activated during puberty.

Most of what we call body odor comes from the armpits. Here there are the special glands that bacteria like, as well as warm moist conditions that are perfect for breeding bacteria. And sweat can get really stinky when bacteria have time to go to work.

Dealing with Perspiration and Body Odor

Puberty changes in body odor and *perspiration* are natural and healthy. It's all a part of growing up. Still, some young people worry about odor and sweating. This isn't really too surprising. Companies spend millions of dollars on TV commercials and magazine ads to make us worry about B.O. and staying "dry." Don't let them make you uptight about your body! Sweating is good for you. It keeps you from frying! It's also your body's way of getting rid of waste products. But there's no reason you have to be smelly even if you sweat a lot.

It's easy to keep yourself smelling clean and fresh. Here are a few tips.

- **Bathe or shower regularly.** Daily washing rinses away the bacteria that cause odor. It's especially important to wash your underarms and genital area.
- **Use an *antibacterial* soap under your arms.** Studies show that these soaps can control bacteria for up to sixteen hours.
- **Wear freshly laundered clothing.** The bacteria that cause odor can hang around in your clothes. Keep them clean.

perspiration (PUR-spuh-RAY-shun)
antibacterial (ann-tee-back-TEER-ee-uhl)

- **Wear clothes that "breathe."** If you perspire quite a bit, try wearing 100 percent cotton underwear. Cotton absorbs more and allows air to circulate, keeping you dry.

Deodorants and Antiperspirants

If the odor or amount of your underarm perspiration bothers you, you may want to use a *deodorant* or an *antiperspirant*. Many deodorants cover up body odor with a scent of their own. Some also fight the bacteria that cause the odor. Antiperspirants keep you dry by cutting down on the amount of perspiration. Most deodorants also contain an antiperspirant.

These products come in sprays, sticks, gels, creams, lotions, and roll-ons. Some are unscented, and some have a scent added. Some are advertised as being especially for men. But there really isn't much difference between a "man's deodorant" and a "woman's deodorant."

Antiperspirants contain some form of *aluminum*. Some experts feel even the small amount of aluminum that could enter the body in this way is unsafe. Other experts say just the opposite. The government sides with those who say it's safe. If you're worried, use a deodorant without aluminum. Or, if you feel you need an antiperspirant, use one with *buffered* aluminum *sulfate*, which isn't easily absorbed beyond the skin's outer layers.

Whatever product you decide to use, do read the directions. Some products should be applied right after

deodorant (dee-OH-der-unt)
antiperspirant (ann-tee-PUR-spuh-runt)
aluminum (uh-LOO-muh-nuhm)
buffered (BUFF-erd)
sulfate (SUL-fate)

you bathe, while you're still damp. Dampness activates the wetness- and bacteria-fighting ingredients. Other products work best when you use them at bedtime rather than first thing in the morning. If you perspire a lot, try using an antiperspirant both before bedtime and before you get dressed in the morning.

PIMPLES AND ACNE

Zits are a fact of life for most boys during puberty. Oil glands in the skin become active—too active. They start working overtime. The extra oil they make often gets trapped behind blocked pores. The result is a faceful of pimples. Sometimes things can get even worse. Then, you've got a full-blown case of acne.

What Causes Acne?

Acne is the term doctors use for what we call zits, pimples, whiteheads, and blackheads. Doctors call all these skin problems acne because they all start with oil glands and clogged pores.

We have oil glands all over our bodies. They are most common on the face, neck, chest, and back. This is also where acne is most likely to strike.

Figure 29 shows a hair follicle and oil gland. Hair follicles lie below the skin's surface. Every hair on your body has its own follicle. In the lower part of each follicle there's an oil gland. These glands make an oil called *sebum*. The sebum flows from the gland and along the hair shaft. It comes out the opening, or pore, in the skin's surface. As the sebum flows out, it carries away dead skin cells from the walls of the hair follicle.

sebum (SEE-bum)

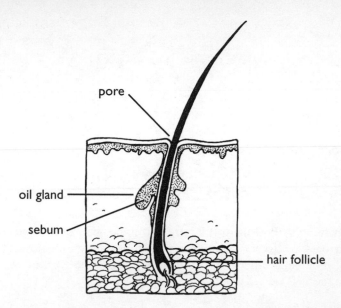

Figure 29. Hair Follicle and Oil Gland. A gland inside the hair follicle makes an oil called sebum. Normally the pore of the hair follicle is unblocked allowing the sebum to slowly flow out and lubricate the skin.

   Puberty affects your hair follicles and oil glands in several ways. The glands make more sebum than ever before. More skin cells come off the wall of the hair follicles. The dead skin cells also tend to stick together more than they did before puberty. These sticky cells can clump together and form a plug that blocks the pore.
   Even though the pore is blocked, the oil gland goes right on making sebum. But the sebum can no longer leave the follicle. It collects behind the plug and swells the hair follicle. This shows up as a white bump just below the skin's surface. We call this white bump a whitehead.

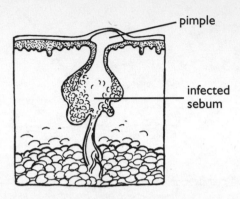

Figure 30. A Pimple. If the pore and upper part of the hair follicle become blocked, the sebum can't flow out through the pore. The result may be an infection in the sebum that results in the swelling and redness we call a pimple.

Sometimes pressure from the trapped sebum pushes the plug up above the skin's surface. If this happens, you develop a blackhead. The black color is not from dirt trapped in the plug. A chemical reaction on the skin's surface turns the plug black.

Whiteheads and blackheads are milder kinds of acne. Pimples are more serious. They occur when bacteria infect the trapped sebum. Bacteria that are harmless when they live on the skin's surface cause the infection. When they get into the sebum trapped behind a blocked pore these "harmless" bacteria begin to multiply. This results in the redness and swelling which we call a pimple. (See Figure 30.)

Sometimes the walls inside an infected hair follicle will burst open. The infection then spreads under the skin. This is the most serious kind of acne. It causes large, painful red bumps.

Treatment

Whiteheads, blackheads, pimples, and severe acne are no fun. They're certainly not very attractive. Worse yet, severe acne can cause permanent pitting or scarring of the skin. The good news is the problem can be treated. In fact, there are a number of things you can do on your own. What works best will depend on the type of acne you have and how severe it is.

Some people think acne is caused by poor hygiene. They think washing more often will cure the problem. This isn't true. Washing your face twice a day is usually enough. Washing more often than that can't prevent or cure acne.

Sometimes oil from the hair can irritate acne breakouts on your forehead. In these cases, washing the hair often and wearing it back, away from the forehead, may help.

Adults may tell you not to pop your pimples. They're right. It can drive the infection deeper into your skin and leave scars.

Over-the-Counter Treatments

"Over-the-counter" means you don't need a doctor's prescription. There are many products you can buy for treating acne. If you use one of these products, there are some things you should know.

- **Benzoyl peroxide.** *Benzoyl peroxide* is the main ingredient in many over-the-counter acne treatments. It attacks the bacteria that cause pimples and acne. It also helps break up the blockage in the pore of

benzoyl peroxide (BEN-zoh-ill) (pur-OCK-side)

ACNE AND FOOD

People used to believe that eating certain foods could cause acne. Chocolate and greasy foods like french fries were the most popular villains. Doctors haven't been able to prove a link between diet and acne. Still, if you find that certain foods give you pimples, it's best to avoid them. You can be sure that eating fewer fried foods and chocolate won't hurt you!

the hair follicle. If you use one of these products, go slow at first. Before using the product, test it on a small area of skin to make sure you're not allergic.

When first using the product, only apply it to the infected area every other day. After a couple of weeks, you can apply it daily. Be careful not to get benzoyl peroxide on your clothes. It's a powerful bleach, which can permanently spot your clothes.

• **Salicylic acid.** *Salicylic acid* is also effective for treating acne. It comes in various over-the-counter products. It removes whiteheads and blackheads and helps prevent their return. Salicylic acid products can be used with other treatments. Follow the directions that come with the product.

• **Abrasive soaps and scrubs.** These can actually make acne worse. Don't use them if you have lots of pimples or severe acne. African-American teenagers should always avoid abrasive soaps or other abrasive products. (See the box on page 113.)

salicylic (sal-uh-SIL-ik)

SPECIAL SKIN CONCERNS
FOR AFRICAN-AMERICANS

African-American men and other men of color need to be especially careful about shaving and treating acne.

- **Abrasive soaps and scrubs.** Abrasive soaps or scrubs can cause permanent patches of lighter or darker skin. Don't use these products.
- **Ingrown hairs.** African-American men may be more likely to develop ingrown hairs. Shaving with a blade razor cuts hair at an angle, leaving a sharp tip. After shaving, curly hair can pull back under the skin's surface or loop over and grow back into the skin (see Figure 31). This can cause irritated, inflamed bumps on the surface of the skin. It's OK to free up the tip of ingrown hair. Don't pluck them, though. Plucking can cause a serious reaction when the hair regrows. If you develop painful razor bumps, lay off shaving for a while. Try an electric instead of a blade razor.
- **Chemical hair removers.** Some men may occasionally use a cream that contains chemical hair removers. Be especially careful if you use one of these products. They can irritate. Always test on a small patch of skin before applying to larger areas. Stay out of the sun and don't go swimming for 24 hours after use.
- **Keloid problems.** African-American skin is more likely to form abnormal scars known as *keloids*. If you're subject to keloids, be especially careful. Even a little nick from shaving or popping a pimple could leave a noticeable scar.

keloids (KEY-loyds)

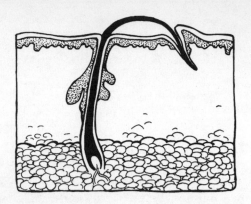

Figure 31. Ingrown Hair

Remember: Any over-the-counter medications for acne may irritate the skin. Always follow the directions carefully. Expect to wait six to eight weeks before seeing results.

Medical Treatment

Some people say, "Just let acne run its course," or "You just have to grow out of it." But medical treatment can help. Also, serious cases of acne can cause permanent scars if left untreated. If you have anything more than mild acne, you may need to see a doctor. The guidelines below will help you decide. See a doctor if you have acne and any of the following are true.

- You have used an over-the-counter product for two months or more, with little or no improvement in your skin.
- Your acne keeps you from fully enjoying your life.
- You have large, red, and painful "acne bumps."

- You are dark-skinned and have noticed that acne is causing dark patches on your skin.
- Severe cases of acne run in your family.
- You are only nine or ten years old when acne first appears.

Your doctor can prescribe a treatment that fits your acne problem. He or she can also prescribe drugs that you can't buy over-the-counter. Always be careful to follow all the directions your doctor gives you. Be sure to tell your doctor about any over-the-counter products you are using or have used in the past. Some products may cause bad interactions with the doctor's prescription. It may take a couple months, or more, of treatment to improve your acne. In some cases your doctor may refer you to a *dermatologist*, a doctor who specializes in skin problems.

Voice Changes

As you go through puberty your voice becomes lower and deeper. This happens because your vocal cords grow thicker and longer, and this changes the tone of your voice. (You can see as well as hear the results of this growth. Your *larynx*, or "voice box," contains the vocal chords and it also grows larger. Boys can see this growth in the larynx as a more pronounced Adam's Apple.) Voice changes usually happen when a boy is about fourteen or fifteen, but, they may happen earlier or later than this. For some boys, this voice change happens without their really noticing it.

dermatologist (DUR-muh-TOL-uh-jist)
larynx (LAR-inks)

I didn't realize that my voice had changed, except that people stopped thinking I was my mom or my sister when I'd answer the phone.

Bill, age 19

For other boys, the change in their voices is more sudden and noticeable.

My throat was sore for about a month or so, kind of scratchy. I thought I just had some kind of sore throat. My voice was kind of froggy. I was always going ahem, ahem— you know, how you clear your throat. Afterward I noticed my voice was deeper than before.

Phil, age 17

As the larynx grows, a boy's voice may "crack." He'll be talking in a normal tone and all of a sudden his voice will get very high and squeaky. This is really embarrassing for many boys. One had this to say:

I'd finally get up my nerve to call a girl on the phone and ask her for a date. I'd say, "Hi, Susie," or whatever her name was, "this is John," and my voice would be just fine. I'd sound perfectly cool. Then I'd say, "Would you like to go to the movies?" And right in the middle my voice would go all high and funny. It would sound like it was Minnie Mouse talking.

John, age 39

Another man said:

Really, it was the most embarrassing thing. It seemed like it happened about all the time. I'd try to control my voice and never get really excited or happy-sounding. Anytime I got nervous and excited, that's when it would happen. I tried not to get too emotional, but of course I did. I never really got control over it. Finally, after a year or maybe it was two years, it stopped happening.

Tyrone, age 28

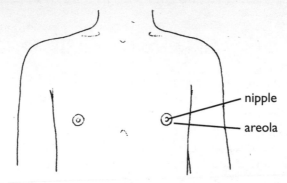

Figure 32. The Areola and Nipple

There's no real reason to be embarrassed. Eventually, your voice will "settle down" and you'll find yourself sounding more adult.

BREAST CHANGES

Breast development—that only happens to girls, right?

Wrong. Boys' breasts don't change as dramatically as girls' do. But they do change. The *areola*, the ring of colored flesh around your nipple, gets wider and darker. (See Figure 32.) The nipple itself gets larger.

Many boys also have some temporary swelling of one or both breasts during puberty. This is a normal change that happens to more than half of the boys going through puberty. The swelling is more noticeable in some boys than in others. In some boys, it's enough to make them worry that they're going to grow breasts and

areola (uh-REE-uh-luh)

THE UPSIDE OF PUBERTY

Puberty isn't all perspiration and pimples. It can seem that way when we've spent a whole class period (or a whole chapter) on the downside. So, at the end of these classes, we remind everybody there's an upside to puberty by listing all the good things that can happen as you go through puberty. Here's one of those lists. What would you add to it?

more privileges
getting to stay out later
being more my own boss
driving a car
getting into R-rated movies
having my body get stronger
more respect
more allowance
joining the team in high school
making my own decisions
   (sometimes)

getting my braces off
getting a job
dating
new school
new friends
going to parties
having my own money
going to college
hanging out with the
   older guys

turn into girls. One man who had quite a bit of breast swelling during puberty told us how he felt.

It was like I was growing breasts. Mine were even bigger than some of the girls'! I got teased about it all the time. I was really afraid that I was turning into a girl. Someone had made this big mistake and I really was a girl. I thought my penis was maybe going to fall off or something. I'd grow breasts and have to wear a bra. I'd heard all sorts of wild stories about boys who turned out to be women and had breasts and penises. But I didn't know anyone I could ask about it.

By the time I was in high school, my chest looked normal. My breasts had gone away. I wish I'd known that it was going to be okay because I really worried about it for a while.

Tom, age 40

Sometimes this swelling makes the breasts feel tender or sore. In addition, there may be a flat button-like bump under one or both nipples. If this happens to you and you don't know that it's perfectly normal, it can be a bit scary. As one man told us:

I had these bumps under my nipples. I thought I had cancer or something.

Harold, age 34

Even though the lumps can be uncomfortable, or even painful, they aren't anything to worry about. It's perfectly normal and not a sign that you have cancer or any other disease. (Men, by the way, only rarely get cancer of the breast, and young boys *never* do.)

The swelling, lumps, and soreness are just a reaction to the new hormones your body is making. Eventually, these problems will go away. This may take a few months or as long as a year and a half. In rare cases, the swelling doesn't go away or it becomes so large that the boy needs medical treatment. Most of the time, though, these breast changes go away on their own.

CHAPTER 6

Changes in the Male Reproductive Organs: Erections, Sperm, and Ejaculation

Having erections is nothing new. Boys have erections long before they start puberty. In fact, males have erections throughout their lives. Even tiny babies still inside their mother's wombs have erections. During puberty, however, boys begin having erections more often than ever before. In this chapter, you'll learn what happens inside your body when you have an erection. You'll also learn about individual differences in erections.

During puberty, a boy's testicles begin to produce ripe sperm. He also ejaculates for the first time. (If you recall from Chapter 1, ejaculation is the release of semen from the opening in the tip of the penis.) In this chapter, you'll learn how your body makes, stores, and releases sperm. You'll learn what happens inside your body when you ejaculate. We'll also talk about the first ejaculation, so you'll know what to expect.

ERECTIONS

The penis responds to sexual stimulation by becoming erect. The stimulation doesn't have to be physical. At times, just *thinking* about sex is enough to cause an erection. But erections aren't always sexual in nature. This is especially true during puberty. You may have erections when you aren't doing or thinking about anything even remotely sexual.

Even with grown men, erections aren't always sexual. For example, a man may wake up in the morning with an erection. Males also have erections while they sleep. These sleep erections happen throughout your life, from the time you're a tiny baby until old age, but they hap-

---

DON'T TAKE OUR WORD FOR IT!

You can find out for yourself what your penis is up to while you sleep. A simple experiment will prove you're having erections during the night. All you need is a strip of postage stamps (not the peel and stick kind).

Before you go to bed, fit a strip of stamps around the shaft of your penis. Bend the stamps back and forth at the perforations once or twice to loosen them up. Don't break the strip, though. Make the strip into a ring that fits snugly around the widest part of the shaft.

The last stamp in your ring should overlap all or part of the first stamp. Moisten the back of the last stamp to make it stick to the first one. Now, go to sleep. Sweet dreams!

Your sleep erections will break the stamp ring apart at the perforations. Wake up and check it out!

pen most often and last longest during puberty. Boys going through puberty average about six or seven erections a night. Each erection usually lasts twenty to thirty minutes.

As you enter puberty, you begin making lots of new hormones. These hormone make your penis especially sensitive. As a result, it often becomes erect. Even when you're not touching it or thinking about sex, bingo . . . suddenly you have an erection. We'll talk more about the erections boys have during puberty and how to cope with them in Chapter 7. First, though, let's look at what happens inside your body during an erection.

The Inside Story

When you have an erection, your penis can get very hard. In fact, an erection is often called a "boner," because at times it may feel like there is a bone in there. There isn't.

There is a lot of spongy *erectile* tissue in your penis. The urethra, the hollow tube that carries urine, runs through the inside of the penis. There are also nerves, blood vessels, and other types of tissue in there; but erectile tissue fills most of the space inside the penis. (See Figure 33.)

Erectile tissue is a spongy mesh of tiny chambers. Normally, the chambers are empty and collapsed flat (like an inner tube that hasn't been blown up). When you get an erection, the vessels carrying blood *into* the penis open wider. Blood rushes in and begins to fill the chambers. As they fill, the spongy tissue swells. The

erectile (ih-REK-tile)

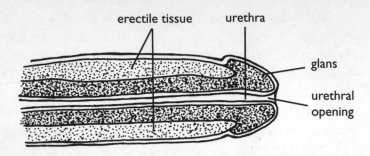

Figure 33. Inside the Penis. The inside of the penis is mostly filled with erectile tissue.

swollen tissue presses against blood vessels in the penis. This slows the flow of blood through the veins leading *out of* the penis.

With more blood coming in and less going out, the tiny chambers soon fill to the max. The erectile tissue becomes swollen with blood. The result: the penis gets hard, rises, and sticks out from your body. You have an erection.

Is Mine Normal?

We get lots of letters from readers asking all sorts of questions about erections. Size questions are, by far, the most common. (Size is discussed in Chapter 3, see pages 48–54.) Readers also ask if it's normal for an erect penis to curve to the left, curve to the right, stand straight up, angle down, or stick straight out. They want to know if their erections happen too often, not often enough, too quickly, or too slowly. They worry that their erections are too soft, too hard, or too . . . whatever!

If you've worried too, fret no more! The list below will give you the facts about normal variations in the erect penis.

Speed: An erection can happen very quickly. In just a matter of seconds, the penis may go from soft and floppy to fully erect. An erection can also happen more slowly. How tired you are, when you last ejaculated, your mood, and whether you've used drugs or alcohol are just a few of the many things that can affect how quickly it gets erect. Age also has a big effect. In general, from puberty onward, the older you get, the longer it takes. But really, what's the rush?

Hardness: Erection is not an all or nothing sort of thing. There are lots of points on the scale between being fully erect and completely soft. Here again, many factors affect how hard an erection is, and again age is a major factor.

Duration: If sexual stimulation continues, a young man may be able to maintain an erection for hours. He won't maintain a full erection for the whole time. Instead, he goes through a repeated cycle from hard to semi-soft to hard again. With a little physical stimulation, a young man may maintain this cycle of erections for hours. The ability to do this also decreases with age.

Curve: When viewed from above, most erections are straight, but there are also many that curve some-what to the left or to the right. When there is a curve, it's usually to the left. Only a small percent-age of males have erections that curve to the right.

Most erections are also straight when viewed from the side. Again, there are also many that curve. If there is a curve, it is usually up (toward the body). Only a small percentage of erect penises curve down (away from the body and toward the floor).

Curves are perfectly normal and quite common, but, if you have a severe curve, or one that causes pain when your penis is erect, check it out with a doctor.

Angle: When you have an erection, your penis sticks out from your body at an angle. Of course, if you're only partly erect, it won't be the same angle as when you're fully erect. However, the angle is usually the same each time you have a full erection. As you can see in Figure 34, the angle of the fully erect penis is different for different men. Some have fairly horizontal erections that stick straight out. Others dip well below the horizon, while still others are nearly vertical. These are all perfectly normal.

Appearance: When your penis is fully erect, it is both longer and wider than when it's soft. The glans, or head, of the penis may get darker in color. Blood vessels on the surface of the penis may be more

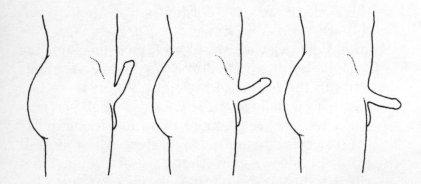

Figure 34. Angle of Erection. The erect penis may stick out at various angles or may stand practically straight up.

noticeable. The skin over these blood vessels may turn blue or darker in color. The urinary opening in the tip of the glans may widen. The testicles may draw up closer to the penis and the rest of the body.

All the variations described above are perfectly normal.

Getting Soft Again

The process of getting soft again is the same if your erection goes away on its own or because you've ejaculated.

First, blood flow *into* the penis slows to normal. This allows blood to begin draining from the spongy tissue and reduces the swelling. Less swelling means less pressure on the blood vessels in the penis. The vessels open up, and more blood flows through the veins leading *out of* the penis.

Once blood flow returns to normal, the extra blood trapped in the erectile tissue drains away. The penis becomes soft and floppy once again.

THE MALE REPRODUCTIVE ORGANS

The sex organs shown in Figure 35 are also called reproductive organs. They allow us to reproduce—to make babies. The male reproductive organs make and deliver sperm. If the sperm unites with an ovum, the female reproductive cell, a baby can grow.

Some male reproductive organs make and store sperm. Others prepare the sperm for ejaculation. Still others provide the routes sperm take as they leave the body during ejaculation. See if you can find the organs listed below in Figure 35.

The Male Reproductive Organs

- **Scrotum:** sac of skin behind the penis that holds the two testicles.
- **Testicles:** two egg-shaped organs; the place where sperm and the hormone testosterone are made.
- **Epididymis:** sperm mature in the *epididymis.*
- **Sperm ducts:** place where mature sperm are stored.
- **Seminal vesicles:** both *seminal vesicles* produce fluid which mixes with sperm and other fluids to make semen.
- **Ejaculatory ducts:** formed by the joining of the sperm ducts and the seminal vesicles, the *ejaculatory ducts* empty into the urethra.
- **Prostate:** here fluids from the *prostate* mix with sperm and other fluids to make semen.
- **Cowper's glands:** a pair of glands just below the prostate on either side of the urethra. They release a small amount of fluid into the urethra before ejaculation.
- **Penis:** external male sex organ that releases semen during ejaculation.
- **Urethra:** tube that runs from the bladder (where urine is stored) along the length of the penis and ends at the urinary opening.
- **Urinary opening:** opening in the tip of the penis.

epididymis (eh-pih-DIH-duh-miss)
seminal vesicles (SEM-in-uhl) (VES-ih-kuhls)
ejaculatory (ih-JACK-you-luh-TOR-ee)
prostate (PRA-state)

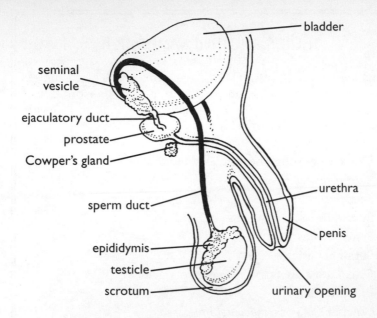

Figure 35. The Male Reproductive Organs

Sperm Factories: The Testicles

The two testicles inside your scrotum are your body's sperm factories. Each testicle is divided into hundreds of little sections. (See Figure 36.) Inside each section are tiny, thread-like tubes. These tubes are coiled *very* tightly. Unwound and stretched out end to end, they'd reach the length of several football fields!

During puberty, a boy begins to make sperm inside these tubes. He usually goes on making fresh sperm every day for the rest of his life. Things may slow down a bit in old age, but, until then, each testicle turns out sperm at a rate of about fifty thousand per minute. Be-

THERE'S ANOTHER NAME FOR IT

In addition to about two jillion slang terms, many of the male reproductive organs also have scientific names. Just in case you're on a quiz show or are planning to be a doctor, we've listed these other terms below.

- **Urinary opening:** the *meatus* or urinary meatus
- **Scrotum:** scrotal sac
- **Testicles:** testes (plural), testis (singular)
- **Sperm ducts:** *vas deferens*, *ductus deferens*
- **Penis:** *phallus*
- **Seminal vesicles**
- **Ejaculatory ducts** } accessory glands
- **Prostate gland**
- **Cowper's glands:** *bulbourethral* glands

tween the two testicles, this comes to six million sperm each hour. Since testicles work around the clock—twenty-four hours a day—that comes to a grand total of 144 million sperm a day! Sperm are alive. When they're fully mature, they look like tadpoles, but real sperm are much smaller than the critter you see in Figure 36. You can't even see a sperm unless you use a microscope. In fact, it would take five hundred sperm, lined up end to end, to cover a distance of one inch!

meatus (me-ATE-us)
vas deferens (vaz DEFF-ih-renz)
ductus deferens (DUCT-us DEFF-ih-renz)
phallus (FAL-us)
bulbourethral (bull-bow-you-REE-thral)

Sperm form in tubes in the testicles. They leave these tubes before they are fully developed. They then mature in a tightly coiled set of tubes, called the *epididymis*. As you can see in Figure 36, the epididymis sits atop and behind the testicle. You have two of them—one for each testicle. You can feel the epididymis. It's the soft and cord-like part you feel at the upper end and back of each testicle. Sperm spend two to six weeks in the epididymis. During those weeks, they develop into mature sperm.

Sperm Storage and Transportation: The Sperm Ducts

Once they're fully developed, sperm move from the epididymis into the sperm ducts. Here again, you have two of them—one for each testicle.

TESTOSTERONE

The testicles do more than make sperm. They also make the "male" hormone testosterone. It's called the "male" hormone because it helps produce sperm and causes many of the changes boys go through during puberty. These changes include the growth of facial hair and muscle tissue, the deepening of the voice, and the broadening of the shoulders. And these are just *some* of the many changes testosterone causes.

The signal that tells your body to make testosterone comes from the brain. Years before you notice any puberty changes, a part of your brain begins to make certain chemicals. These chemicals travel to the pituitary gland at the base of the brain. They cause the pituitary to make certain hormones, which travel through the bloodstream to the testicles. They cause the testicles to make a hormone of their own: testosterone. Though it's called the male hormone, females, too, make testosterone in their bodies, but only in small amounts.

Sperm ducts are one and a half to two feet in length. They begin in the scrotum and continue up into the main part of the body. In Figure 35, you can see how the ducts run up into the body and loop around the bladder.

Mature sperm are stored in the sperm ducts until they leave the body during ejaculation, or until they die. If a male doesn't ejaculate for a while, the sperm soon die and are absorbed by the body. Millions more are produced every day to replace the ones that die.

When a male ejaculates, muscles in the walls of the sperm ducts contract. These contractions pump the sperm up into the body where they mix with other fluids to become semen.

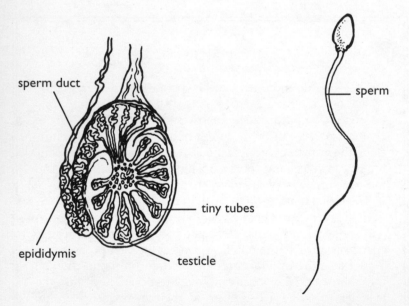

Figure 36. Inside the Testicle. Sperm are made in tiny tubes inside the testicle. They mature in the epididymis and are stored in the sperm duct.

Sperm Plus Prostate and Seminal Fluids Equals Semen

Look at Figure 35. You can see one of the seminal vesicles at the base of the bladder. (There are actually two seminal vesicles, one on each side.) You can also see the prostate just below the seminal vesicle. (There is only one doughnut-shaped prostate.) Each seminal vesicle connects with one of the two sperm ducts, inside the prostate, where it forms one of the two ejaculatory ducts. These one-inch long tubes lie within the prostate and empty into the urethra. During ejaculation, semen is formed when sperm mix with fluids from the seminal vesicles and prostate in the ejaculatory ducts. It is semen—not just sperm—that comes out of the penis when you ejaculate. "Cum" is a slang word for semen.

On the average, a little less than a teaspoon of semen comes out of the penis when a man ejaculates. There are 300–500 million sperm in this small amount of fluid. Remember, though, sperm are very tiny. They are only a small part of the semen you ejaculate. Most of the fluid comes from the seminal vesicles and prostate.

Tubes, Tubes, and More Tubes

Inside the prostate, the ejaculatory ducts empty into the urethra. The urethra is another tube. (Seems like you're just full of tubes, doesn't it?) Its upper end connects to the bladder, the place where urine (pee) is stored. The urethra then passes through the prostate and into the penis. It runs the whole length of the penis and its lower end forms the urinary opening in the tip of the penis.

When you ejaculate, semen is pumped through the urethra and out the urinary opening. When you pee, urine also travels through the urethra and leaves the body through the same urinary opening.

GATORADE FOR SPERM

Football players drink Gatorade during a game because it's packed full of sugar and vitamins. It gives the players an instant energy boost. Fluid from the seminal vesicles is like Gatorade for sperm. It is very powerful stuff, full of nutrients and rich in sugar, for quick energy. If it weren't for this sperm Gatorade, we wouldn't be here. Without the energy boost it gives, a sperm would not be able to reach a woman's ovum and fertilize it.

After all, from the penis to the ovum is a very long journey for the tiny sperm. After being ejaculated from the penis, the sperm must first swim to the top of the vagina. Then, they must pass through the cervix, the narrow tunnel that leads to the uterus. Next, they have to travel the whole length of the uterus. Finally, the sperm have to swim halfway up the uterine tube to find the ovum.

There are millions of sperm, but only one can enter the ovum and fertilize it. That's a lot of competition! The winning sperm must swim very fast, indeed, to beat all the others to the ovum.

Altogether, sperm have to travel about six inches. This doesn't sound like much, but, sperm are less than one five-hundredth of an inch long. Six inches to a sperm would be like three miles to you or me. Wouldn't you need an energy boost if you were going to run three miles at top speed?

"Oh, gross . . . totally disgusting!"That's what my students (the girls at least) say when they realize urine and semen use the same route to exit the body. But there's nothing gross or disgusting about it. Urine is just another liquid. Unless you have an infection, your urine is germ-free. Semen is perfectly clean, too.

Besides, semen and urine don't travel through the urethra at the same time. When you're about to ejaculate, the connection between the bladder and the ure-thra closes. Urine can't leave the bladder, and semen can't get into the bladder.

Sperm are sensitive to urine. This is one reason the body prevents semen and urine from travelling through the urethra at the same time. To make sure that sperm aren't damaged by urine, your body rinses the urethra with a special fluid. Before you ejaculate, the Cowper's glands release a small amount of this fluid, called *pre-ejaculatory* fluid. This fluid neutralizes any leftover traces of urine that may be left in the urethra. We'll talk more about pre-ejaculatory fluid as we explain ejaculation.

EJACULATION

Doctors, it seems, just can't resist dividing things into stages. They've divided the ejaculation into two stages: *emission* and *expulsion*. In the emission stage, sperm and other fluids are mixed together to form semen. The ex-pulsion stage is the actual ejaculation of the semen from the penis (see Figure 37). Altogether both stages of ejac-ulation last only about ten seconds or so. The feelings are so intense, though, that it often seems longer.

Emission

This stage begins with muscle contractions in the prostate, seminal vesicles, testicles, epididymis, and sperm ducts. The contractions pump sperm upward out of the sperm ducts into the ejaculatory ducts. At the same time, contractions squeeze fluids out of the semi-

pre-ejaculatory (PREE-ih-JACK-you-luh-TOR-ee)
emission (ee-MIH-shun)
expulsion (x-PULL-shun)

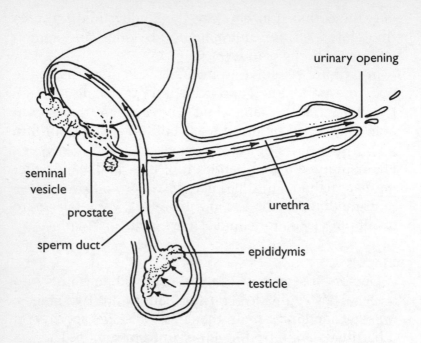

Figure 37. Semen and Ejaculation. Shortly before ejaculation, muscles in each testicle, epididymis, and sperm duct contract rhythmically. Sperm are pumped up through the sperm ducts into the main part of the body and into the prostate. In the ejaculatory duct the sperm mix with fluid from the seminal vesicles and prostate to form semen. At the time of ejaculation, more muscle contractions pump the semen through the urethra and out the urinary opening.

nal vesicles and the prostate. Inside the ejaculatory ducts these fluids mix with the sperm. As we know, this mixture of sperm and fluids from the seminal vesicles and prostate is called semen. Contractions then pump the semen into the top of the urethra. During this stage, the connection with the bladder closes off, so semen and urine can't mix.

Just before and during the emission stage, the feeling of sexual excitement is building very quickly. Once emission occurs, you know for sure that the ejaculation is coming and can't be stopped.

Expulsion

During the second stage of ejaculation, semen is forced from the upper urethra by a series of contractions. Powerful muscle contractions push the semen along the length of the penis. The semen then comes out the opening in the tip of the penis in spurts.

The first three or four contractions are the strongest. They occur a little less than a second apart. They force most of the semen out of the penis in three or four spurts. Weaker and less regular contractions may continue for several seconds. They gently push out any remaining semen.

The contractions may be so strong that the semen shoots a distance of a foot or more, but the force of the contractions varies from one time to the next and also from one person to the next. Rather than shooting, the semen may ooze or dribble out. Your age and other factors—including how long it has been since you last ejaculated—may affect the force of the contractions.

About a teaspoon or so of semen comes out of the penis during ejaculation. The amount varies. If a male hasn't ejaculated for a while, there's likely to be more semen than if he's ejaculated recently. The color also varies. It may be white, off-white, grayish, or clear. Sometimes, it has a yellowish or orange tinge to it.

When a grown man's semen is first released, it's often thick, like a gel. Within five to twenty-five minutes, it becomes liquid. Scientists believe the gel-like state helps the sperm survive inside a woman's body.

As it dries on the skin, semen may be a little flaky. It may leave a stain on cloth. It may also make the cloth a bit stiff as it dries.

Like the color, the consistency of semen varies. It isn't always thick and gel-like. Sometimes it creamy or more watery. It may be rather sticky.

Pre-Ejaculatory Fluid

Sometimes, a drop or two of a clear or slightly cloudy, sticky fluid appears at the tip of the penis before ejaculation. This is the pre-ejaculatory fluid made by Cowper's glands. A slang term for this fluid is pre-cum. As we said, this fluid flushes out the urethra. It neutralizes any acids from urine that could harm the sperm.

Pre-ejaculatory fluid may appear during the emission stage or earlier. Sometimes it appears soon after a male becomes aroused and gets an erection. Usually, there's only a drop or two. Sometimes, though, there's quite a bit more—more like ten or twenty drops. The longer the time between erection and ejaculation, the more of this fluid there's likely to be.

You may not see it every time you ejaculate. In fact, some men rarely, if ever, notice any of this fluid. Visible, or not, the release of pre-ejaculatory fluid is a normal part of the sexual excitement.

Pre-ejaculatory fluid may contain live sperm. (This is one reason why a woman can get pregnant even if her male partner pulls out of her vagina before he ejaculates.)

The First Ejaculation

The age at which boys start making sperm and ejaculate for the first time varies greatly from one boy to the next. Some boys ejaculate very early in puberty. Their testicles have hardly begun to grow and they have little or no pubic hair. On the other hand, some boys don't start to ejaculate until they reach Stage 5 of both pubic hair and genital growth.

Most boys ejaculate for the first time when they are between the ages of eleven and fifteen and a half, but there are also some boys who ejaculate when they are younger or older than this. Most boys have their first ejaculation when they masturbate or have a wet dream. *Masturbation* is rubbing, stroking, or otherwise stimulating your sex organs to give yourself sexual pleasure. A wet dream is an ejaculation that happens while you're asleep. We'll explain more about masturbation and wet dreams in the next chapter, but, at this point, we should probably explain the difference between ejaculation and *orgasm*. Ejaculation is the physical act of releasing semen from the penis. Orgasm is the sensation, or feeling, that usually accompanies ejaculation. It is a spasm of intense sexual pleasure that occurs when the tension that builds during sexual excitement is suddenly released.

Ejaculation and orgasm usually go together, but it is possible to have one without the other. For example, many boys have orgasms before they reach puberty. By definition, however, they don't ejaculate until they begin to make sperm. Remember, ejaculation is the release of semen and semen is a mixture of sperm and other fluids. If you aren't making sperm yet, you certainly can't release semen that contains them. (You'll learn more about orgasms in Chapter 7.)

At first, a boy's semen may contain very few sperm.

masturbation (MASS-tur-BAY-shun)
orgasm (OR-gaz-um)

The sperm he does have are not always the fully mature type that are capable of fertilizing an ovum. It may take a couple of years before a boy is ejaculating a sizable number of fully mature sperm, but even early on he may ejaculate *some* mature sperm. So, once a boy ejaculates for the first time, he is considered capable of fathering a child. (This doesn't, of course, mean he's ready to be a parent, just that he's *physically* capable of being one.)

At first, a boy may ejaculate semen that tends to be clear or slightly yellow or orange. As a boy grows older and begins making a larger amount of mature sperm, his ejaculations will probably be more whitish in color. As a boy matures, the force of the contractions that pump out his semen during an ejaculation increases. In younger boys semen often dribbles or oozes out. As they get older, it is more likely to shoot out, though this isn't always the case. Whether the semen oozes or shoots out has no affect whatsoever on the ability to father a child.

Before we leave this discussion of the male reproductive organs, we want to talk about some common and not-so-common medical problems.

THE MALE REPRODUCTIVE ORGANS: HEALTH ISSUES

Boys often ask questions about health issues and medical problems that affect their reproductive organs. For this reason, we decided to include some relevant information in the book. But the following information should not alarm you. It should make you alert, not paranoid.

Cancer of the Testicles and TSE

Cancer of the testicles is the most common type of cancer in males aged fifteen to thirty-five. It kills more

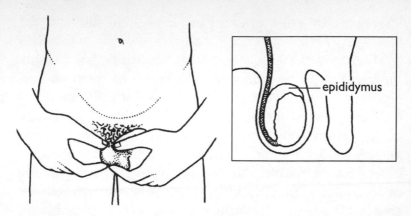

epididymus

Figure 38. Testicular Self-Exam. A testicular self-exam should be done once each month. Both hands should be used to examine each testicle.

young men than any other type of cancer. However, it is very curable if found and treated at an early stage.

Examining your testicles once a month can literally save your life. It allows you to detect the very earliest warning sign of cancer of the testicles—a small lump in one of the testicles. In the early stages, there are usually no symptoms other than a lump. Often only one testicle is affected. The lump is usually painless. However, some men do have a heaviness or a dull ache. The best way to protect yourself is to find the cancer early on, by doing a monthly *testicular* self-exam (TSE). Also have an exam done by your doctor at your regular check-ups. Self exams and medical exams are particularly important for anyone who has, or once had, an undescended testicle. (See pages 69 to 71.) An undescended testicle, even if

testicular (tes-TICK-you-lar)

it's been corrected, puts a person at increased risk for testicular cancer.

The American Academy of Family Physicians recommends that all boys between the ages of thirteen and eighteen learn to do TSE. Since TSE should be done once a month, some men always do TSE on the first day of the month in order to make it easy to remember. Like all new things, TSE takes some practice, but, once you've been doing it awhile, the exam only takes three minutes or so. Ideally, TSE should be done after a warm bath or shower. The heat causes the scrotal skin to relax, making it easier to feel anything unusual on the testicle. The exam should be done while you're sitting or lying down.

Check one testicle at a time. Be sure to always check both because often only one is affected. Use both hands to examine each testicle. Place the index and middle fingers underneath the testicle, and the thumbs on top (see Figure 38). Roll the testicle gently between the thumbs and fingers. It should feel smooth and firm but not hard. (Remember: One testicle is slightly larger than the other. Don't worry. That's normal.)

You will feel a soft, cord-like structure on the top and back of the testicles. This is not an abnormal lump. It's the epididymis. Gently separate it from the testicle with your fingers and feel the testicle itself. You're looking for a lump which is usually the size of a pea. It may feel like a piece of gravel or a peanut.

If you do find a lump, it doesn't mean you have cancer. The lump may be due to an infection, but you should call your doctor right away because any lump needs to be examined. If it is due to an infection, your doctor can decide on the proper treatment. If the lump is cancerous, there are excellent treatments for that, too. Remember that testicular cancer is highly curable, especially when detected and treated early.

Pain in the Testicles

Almost every boy knows the severe pain that can accompany an accidental blow to the testicles. It is also possible to experience sudden and severe testicular pain even when there is no injury. Here's some information to help you deal with both these situations.

Severe Pain Following Injury: Because they hang down outside of the body, the scrotum and testicles are subject to injury. Any blow to these parts can cause severe pain, but most accidental injuries do not require medical treatment.

If you receive a blow to the testicles, apply cold compresses or an ice bag. Lie down so there's no strain on the scrotum or testicles. If the pain starts to ease within an hour or so, you can assume no serious damage has been done.

However, call your doctor or go to the emergency room right away if any of the following happens:
- the pain doesn't begin to let up within an hour or so
- the pain gets worse
- there's bruising or swelling
- you have difficulty urinating or have bloody (pinkish) urine

Any of the above could mean there's bleeding inside the testicle or scrotum. If left untreated, healthy tissue could be damaged. So, if you have any of the above symptoms, call your doctor or go to the emergency room right away.

JOCKSTRAPS AND OTHER
ATHLETIC SUPPORTERS

Injuries to the scrotum and testicles can be *very* painful. To protect yourself during contact sports, use a cup protector. The cup fits over the penis and scrotum. It is held in place by a jockstrap (see Figure 39). The soft cup type is recommended for soccer. For high impact sports like football or boxing, you need the hard plastic cup.

Boys often worry about what size to buy. Jockstrap sizes do not refer to the size of your sex organs. Jockstraps are sold by *waist* size. Different brands scale sizes differently. Ignore the "small," "medium," or "large." Look for the waist size in inches, which will be printed somewhere on the label. Cups come in two sizes: adult and youth (for boys).

For sports that involve running, jumping, and sudden movement, you can wear a jockstrap without a cup or some other type of athletic supporter. The supporter tucks the scrotum and testicles up close to the body to protect them from jarring. Jockstraps are not all that comfortable. Many athletes are turning to other types of supporters. Running shorts combine outer shorts with an inner "hammock" to hold your genitals. Compression shorts squeeze everything into a special type of two-layer shorts. The outer shorts are usually nylon mesh. The inner shorts fit tightly and are made from a stretchable material like Spandex® or Lycra®.

It's important to wash your athletic supporter often. Otherwise you might end up with a fungus infection, sometimes known as "jock itch" or "jock rot."

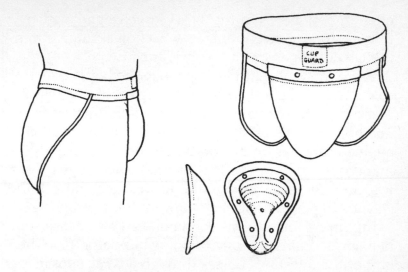

Figure 39. Jockstrap and Cup Protector

Some injuries can be prevented by wearing a jockstrap or some other type of athletic supporter during sports activities (see box, page 144).

Sudden, Severe Pain Without Injury: See your doctor or go to the emergency room immediately, if you have sudden, severe pain in a testicle without an injury to explain the pain. Even if the pain disappears as suddenly as it appeared, you still need immediate medical care. The two most likely causes of this type of pain are *torsion* (twisting) and *inguinal hernia*.

Testicular Torsion: This is an uncommon but serious, extremely painful condition in which the testicle becomes twisted within the scrotum. It happens most

torsion (TOR-shin)
inguinal hernia (ING gwuh nuhl) (HER-nee-uh)

often in boys between the ages of twelve and eighteen. It may follow strenuous exercise or lifting. Often, though, it happens with no obvious cause.

The symptoms may develop while the boy is asleep. If so, he may wake to sudden, severe pain in one testicle. There may be swelling, nausea and vomiting, or fever. The boy may feel faint. The condition requires immediate medical care. Time is of the essence to prevent permanent damage or the loss of the testicle. Even if the testicle returns to normal, the testicle may have to be stitched in place surgically to prevent future problems.

Inguinal Hernia: This condition can also cause sudden severe pain in the scrotum. A hernia occurs when part of the intestines bulges through a weak spot in the wall of the abdomen. If it happens in the lower part of the abdomen, it can cause pain and a bulge in the scrotum. If untreated, hernias can cause serious medical problems. But, if treated promptly, they are not serious. The treatment usually consists of an operation to repair the weak spot.

Luckily these medical problems are not very common. It's good to know something about them, but, if you're like most boys, you'll be more interested in the next chapter, which talks about masturbation and orgasms.

CHAPTER 7

Spontaneous Erections, Orgasms, Masturbation, and Wet Dreams

Erections happen in response to touching and other forms of sexual stimulation. In Chapter 6, you learned that males also have erections during sleep. They may also have erections even though they're wide awake and aren't doing—or even thinking about—anything sexual. These are called *spontaneous* erections. They occur particularly often during puberty.

Spontaneous refers to the fact that these erections happen "all by themselves," without touching or other sexual stimulation. *Reflex, involuntary,* or unwanted erections are other names for these erections. In this chapter, you'll learn about spontaneous erections and how to cope with them.

In Chapter 6 you also learned about orgasms—the physical feelings of sexual pleasure that usually go with ejaculation. In this chapter, you'll learn more about or-

spontaneous (spon-TAY-nee-us)
reflex (REE-flex)
involuntary (in-vol-uhn-TEAR-ee)

gasms and how your body responds when you are sexually aroused ("turned on").

As we explained in Chapter 6, most boys have their first ejaculation while masturbating. Masturbating means touching, stroking, rubbing, or otherwise stimulating your genitals for sexual pleasure. Some boys ejaculate for the first time during a wet dream. Wet dreams are ejaculations that happen while you're asleep. If you're like most boys, you probably have a lot of questions about masturbation and wet dreams. We'll try to answer those questions in this chapter.

SPONTANEOUS ERECTIONS

Getting erections easily and often is a fact of life during puberty. It takes a while for your penis to get used to all the new sex hormones your body is making. Your penis is supersensitive. But as you get older, your penis won't be so quick to jump to attention, and you'll have spontaneous erections less often. Meanwhile, they can be embarrassing. One boy in my class told this story:

> I was on the beach wearing my BVs. [BVs are low-cut bathing suits made from thin nylon.] I saw this really curvy girl lying on her towel. My penis got hard and I had to run into the ocean so no one would see.
>
> *Darryl, age 12*

Another boy said:

> Yeah, I get erections sometimes when I'm out running. That's how come I always wear a pair of gym shorts over my sweatpants. You get a hard-on and it sticks out like a tent pole in those baggy sweats.
>
> *Julio, age 13*

One man remembered how it was for him:

> It would happen at any time. I'd be at school, standing in the hall or something, and bingo, I'd have a hard-on. I'd shuffle my school books around and try and hold them in front of me so no one could see. It was really embarrassing.
>
> *Joe, age 32*

Many told stories about getting erections when they had to get up in front of the class.

> I had to give a speech one time in public-speaking class. I had this really funny speech, and I'm standing there doing it and I get this big hard-on. I didn't know if everyone was laughing at my speech or at my hard-on.
>
> *Tyrone, age 28*

If you're having spontaneous erections more often, it helps to know that they're perfectly normal. Remember,

---

COPING WITH ERECTIONS

You can't stop them from happening. Here's some advice to help you cope, though.

- Wear long shirts and let them hang out over your pants.
- Shift your notebook to cover your erection.
- Carry a book to hold in front of your erection.
- Sit down when you get an erection.
- Put your hands in your pants pockets and shift your penis to the side.
- Wear a sweatshirt tied around your waist so that the sleeves cover your front.
- Think about something else until it goes away.

---

you're not the only one. Other boys your age are going through the same thing. Remember, too, your erection isn't as obvious to others as it is to you.

ORGASM

Orgasm is the sudden, explosive release of sexual tension that usually accompanies ejaculation. It is possible to have an orgasm without ejaculating. For example, boys often masturbate to the point of orgasm before they reach puberty and begin ejaculating. It's also possible to ejaculate without experiencing an orgasm. Usually, though, ejaculation and orgasm happen together.

It's difficult to describe *exactly* what an orgasm feels like. Orgasms vary from person to person and from time to time for the same person. Sometimes your orgasm may be very strong, with pleasurable feelings starting in the genitals and radiating to the whole body. At other times, your orgasm may be less intense, and the feeling remains centered in the genital area, but, however many differences there are, men's general descriptions of their orgasms are often quite similar.

Men often describe their orgasms as beginning with a feeling of deep warmth or pressure. This corresponds to the emission stage of ejaculation. During this stage, contractions force semen into the upper urethra (see Chapter 6, page 136).

There is also the feeling that orgasm and ejaculation are coming and can't be stopped. Then, there are sharp, intensely pleasurable contractions in the whole genital area. Some men describe this as a pumping sensation. Finally, there's a warm rush of fluid or a shooting sensation as the semen travels through the urethra and is ejaculated out the urinary opening.

Both emotional and physical factors affect the intensity of the orgasm. The amount of semen ejaculated may be one factor. You ejaculate more semen than usual if you have gone without ejaculating for a while. Your orgasm is usually more intense, too. On the other hand, if you ejaculate more than once in a short period of time, there will be less semen each time. The intensity of the orgasms usually also decreases. An orgasm only lasts for a matter of seconds. But the feeling is so intense that it may seem much longer.

Some of the men we interviewed describe orgasms as "great," "terrific," or "beautiful." Some said, "There's just no words to describe it," or "It's not something you can explain." Some men, however, were able to describe it in detail. One man gave a description that other men agreed was pretty good. Here's what he said:

> Well, it feels like there's a sort of neat sensation in my genitals and body that builds up and then goes off, a sort of wave of good sensual feeling throughout the whole body. The spurting part, when the semen is actually coming out, is a jerky kind of thing. It's not really all that great a feeling, but the waves of the sensual feeling are timed with pulses of the spurt, which does feel great. Afterward, I feel tingling and then relaxed all over.
>
> *Will, age 46*

The Male Sexual Response

Orgasm is the peak of the body's response to sexual arousal (being "turned on"). The changes in the male body leading to and following orgasm—as well as the orgasm itself—are called the male sexual response. Sometimes the response is more intense than at other times, but it's basically the same whether you're masturbating by yourself or having sex with a partner.

The male sexual response begins with sexual *arousal* and erection. The erection may last until after orgasm. Or it may decrease and increase a number of times before ejaculation actually takes place.

As arousal continues and builds toward orgasm, several other changes take place. The skin of the scrotum gets thicker and tighter. The testicles begin to swell and draw up closer to the body. By the time you reach orgasm, the testicles may have increased as much as 50 percent in size.

Muscle tension increases as sexual excitement builds. Heart rate and blood pressure increase, too. Breathing becomes deeper and heavier. The skin on the face, chest or other parts of the body may get flushed and red or deeper in color. This is called the sex flush. The nipples may get stiff and stand out more. The muscles around the anus tighten. The opening in the head, or glans, of the penis widens. The glans of the penis may swell and darken in color. A drop or two of pre-ejaculatory fluid may appear at the tip of the penis.

Sexual arousal may continue to build to the point of orgasm or may stop before then. If it continues, the heart rate and muscle tension also continue to increase, and the feelings of sexual excitement grow stronger.

As orgasm is about to happen, there is a feeling of building to a climax. Muscle tension and heart rate reach their maximum. During orgasm, there is an explosive release of the tension that has been building in the muscles. Waves of muscle contractions in the genital area give feelings of intense physical pleasure. The contractions happen a little less than a second apart. The first

arousal (uh-ROW-zuhl)

three or four are the strongest and give the most intense pleasure.

At the point of orgasm, there may be involuntary muscle movements in the face (a grimace) or the hands and feet (clutching, grasping, arching). There may be muscle spasms in other parts of the body as well.

After orgasm, the body relaxes and begins to return to normal. Some men perspire heavily at this point, even if they haven't exerted themselves a great deal, but heart rate, breathing, and blood pressure all return to normal. The testicles and scrotum loosen up. The penis gets soft again. It may take anywhere from five minutes to two hours for the body to completely return to normal.

After an orgasm, men often feel very relaxed, and they may be sleepy. There is a period of time during which they cannot have another orgasm, even though they may have a partial or full erection. This period of time may last for a matter of minutes to a day or more. Generally, the older a man gets, the more time it takes before he's ready for another orgasm.

You may not be aware of all the changes we've been describing. The feelings of physical pleasure that come with these changes can be very intense. You may get too caught up in what you're feeling to notice all the details.

MASTURBATION

As we've said, masturbation means "deliberate touching or stroking of the sex organs for sexual pleasure." Slang terms include "jacking off," "playing with yourself," "beating your meat," "doing it," and "pulling the joystick." You've probably heard a lot of other ones, too.

If a man or boy masturbates long enough, he usually has an orgasm, but he may stop masturbating before he gets to that point. Or, if he's just recently had an orgasm, he may not be able to have another one right away. Even if he doesn't have an orgasm, though, his erection will still go away after a while.

Most boys (and men, too) masturbate. Not all do, though. It's normal if you do and normal if you don't. A boy can masturbate to orgasm before he begins to go through puberty, but he won't ejaculate.

Some males start to masturbate when they're kids and continue throughout their lives. Some don't masturbate until they start puberty and begin making sperm. These boys may have their first orgasm and their first ejaculation at the same time. Some don't start until they're older. And there are some who never masturbate.

However, the large majority of males do masturbate. In one survey, 95 percent of males and 89 percent of females reported masturbating. Yes, females masturbate, too! In fact, people of all ages, both sexes, and all walks of life masturbate. Of course, females don't ejaculate sperm like men do, but they do have orgasms. Some women also produce a sudden gush of fluid just as they're having an orgasm, but this is not an ejaculation of the same type men have.

Boys sometimes have the idea that once you start having sex, you stop masturbating. Not true. Many married people and others with steady sex partners masturbate, even if they're having intercourse regularly.

You Don't See Any Blind, Crazy, Morons Around Here, Do Ya?

People used to think that all sorts of horrible things would happen if you masturbated. You'd grow warts on your nose and hair on the palms of your hands, go insane or blind, suffer heart attacks, pimples, wet and clammy hands, blindness, softening of the brain, idiocy, and insanity (to mention just a few). Nowadays, we know that none of these things is true. (If they were, there would be an awful lot of blind, insane idiots around.)

People no longer believe these old stories, but the idea that masturbation might be harmful still lingers on. So, just in case you've heard some of the modern myths about masturbation, we'd like to tell you the real facts.

You won't "run out of" or "use up" all your sperm because of masturbating. You might temporarily reduce your sperm supply by repeated ejaculations. But as you know from reading this book, your body is constantly making millions of new sperm each day. There's just no way you could run out.

Masturbating a lot when you're young will not have harmful effects on your adult sex life. Some boys worry that if they masturbate a whole lot when they're young, they'll learn to like it so much that they won't enjoy sexual intercourse. Or, they think the penis will get "too used to" masturbation and it won't be possible to ejaculate inside the vagina. Or, they're worried that masturbation will make the penis too sensitive or too insensitive to work properly during intercourse. The theories go on and on . . . and they're all wrong.

Things just don't work that way. In fact, most experts agree that masturbating is a way of rehearsing for your adult sex life. By masturbating, you learn how your own body responds and what gives you the most pleasure. When you do begin to have sex, you'll know more about what you like, about what "turns you on." If you know this about yourself, it's that much easier to tell your sex partner what you like and don't like and how your partner can help increase your sexual pleasure.

Some men have more physically intense orgasms from masturbation than from intercourse. This doesn't necessarily mean that they *like* masturbation more than intercourse. Intercourse involves touching, holding, and being intimate with another person. That makes it a very different kind of experience than masturbating.

Other men find that the orgasms they experience during intercourse are more intense than those they have during masturbation. Still others don't find any difference in intensity.

As you grow older, you may find that masturbating provides the most intense orgasms, that sexual intercourse does, or that the intensity is the same with both. How much or how little you masturbate when you're young won't have anything to do with what type of orgasms are most intense for you when you're an adult.

Remember, masturbation is not in any way harmful.

If you masturbate and ejaculate a whole lot, your penis might get sore from all the rubbing. But other than this soreness, masturbating cannot hurt your body.

• No, you're not masturbating too much. How do I know? Well, of course I have no idea how much you're masturbating, but your body sets it own limits. If a boy masturbates a great deal, his penis just won't get erect for a while. He'll have to give it a rest before he can get an erection again.

I suppose I should qualify my statement a little. If you're masturbating so much that it's all you do, if you never go anywhere, don't have any friends, don't have any hobbies or interests other than masturbating, and spend all your free time alone in your room masturbating . . . OK, yeah, you're masturbating too much. Short of that, you're fine.

Some boys masturbate several times a day. Some do it once or twice a day. Some once or twice a week. Some boys masturbate more often or less often than this, and some never masturbate. All are normal.

Sexual Fantasies

Many people like to imagine things that make them feel more excited as they masturbate. Imagining or pretending that something is happening is called daydreaming or fantasizing. We daydream and *fantasize* about all sorts of things. We might, for instance, daydream about being a major league football player or a rock star. When our daydreams are about sexual things, we call them sexual *fantasies*.

Almost everyone has sexual fantasies. We may have them while we're masturbating and at other times, too. Sexual fantasies can be a rich and varied way of experimenting with your sexual self. Sometimes, the things we fantasize about are things we might actually like to do someday. Other times we fantasize about things that we'd feel embarrassed or even bad about if we actually did them.

Some people worry that there might be something weird about their sexual fantasies. If you've ever been concerned about this, you can relax. Human beings (both males and females) have sexual fantasies about all sorts of things. If you think you're the only one who's ever had a particular fantasy—you're wrong. We guaran-

fantasies (FAN-tuh-sees)
fantisize (FAN-tuh-size)

tee that there are plenty of other people who've had almost that exact same fantasy. Still, if you're disturbed by the type of fantasies you're having, you should talk this over with a therapist or counselor. See the Resource Section (pages 226–227) for information on finding someone to talk to.

FAQs (Frequently Asked Questions)

The boys in my classes always have a lot of questions about masturbation. Here are answers to some of the questions they ask most frequently.

Can masturbation affect your athletic performance?
There is no evidence to suggest that masturbation affects your athletic ability. It could even be possible that masturbating might help you relax before the big game.

Is masturbation "sinful" or morally wrong?
One person's idea of what's "sinful" or morally wrong may be quite different from another person's. Nowadays, most people do not think masturbation is morally wrong or sinful, and personally, we go along with that point of view. In the past, many religions held that masturbation was a sin. Many religious leaders no longer feel this way, but some still do. For example, the Catholic religion's official point of view holds that masturbation is a sin. This doesn't mean that all Catholics or even all Catholic priests and church leaders feel this way.
If you're bothered by the notion that masturbation may be sinful or morally wrong, perhaps you should talk with your minister, priest, or religious leader.

Is it weird for a boy to masturbate with other boys?
Some boys learn about masturbation from other boys.

Some boys even experiment by masturbating together. Boys who do this often worry about whether this is weird. Sometimes they think that this means that they are *homosexual*.

Homosexuals are people who prefer to have sexual contacts with people who are the same sex as they are. Most adults in our society are *heterosexuals*. Heterosexuals are people who prefer to have sexual experiences with people of the opposite sex. We'll talk more about homosexuality in Chapter 9. For now you should know that masturbating with other boys does not mean you are a homosexual. Many boys engage in some form of what we call "sex play" with other boys as they're growing up. You may have had such experiences and have wondered about them or felt uncomfortable. If so, be sure to read Chapter 9, where we talk more about these things.

I was masturbating and I didn't want to get semen all over my pajamas, so I put my finger over the top of my penis just as I was ejaculating so nothing would come out. And nothing did, but for the last couple of days I've had this pain in my penis and this milky stuff has come out. What should I do?

This kind of problem sometimes happens. It's called *retrograde* ejaculation. It happens when the semen is prevented from spurting out through the opening at the tip of the penis. In older men, there are certain medical problems that cause retrograde ejaculation, but in boys, it usually happens when the boy is masturbating, and doesn't want the semen to come out.

homosexual (ho-mo-SEK-shoo-uhl)
heterosexuals (HET-er-oh-SEK-shoo-uhls)
retrograde (RET-row-grade)

Retrograde means "going backward." In retrograde ejaculation, the semen can't come out the end of the penis, so it travels backward in the urethra. It may be forced up the tube that leads to the bladder. As a result the urine may be cloudy for some time. The semen may also be forced into the prostate. In either case, there may be pain and discharge from the penis.

In some cases, the symptoms will clear up all by themselves, but often a doctor's care is needed. Although it may be embarrassing to explain how the retrograde ejaculation happened, it's important to see the doctor if you have pain, a milky discharge, or milky urine. The prostate can become irritated and susceptible to infection if semen is forced up into it. The doctor can treat such infections with antibiotics. If necessary, he can give you painkillers. To avoid these medical problems, let your semen come out normally.

When I make out with my girlfriend for a long time, I end up with an achy feeling in my testicles. Why does this happen?

This condition is sometimes called "blue balls" or "lover's nuts." When you get sexually excited, your penis gets erect and also your testicles are filled with extra blood. When a man ejaculates, blood vessels open and blood flows rapidly through the veins leading out of his penis and testicles. Without an ejaculation, this rapid release of blood doesn't occur. The result can be an achy, uncomfortable feeling in the testicles. This is not a harmful condition. Masturbation may relieve the achy feeling.

If a boy doesn't masturbate or have sexual intercourse, what happens to all the sperm?

If a boy doesn't ejaculate through masturbation or intercourse, one of two things may happen. The sperm die and are reabsorbed by the body. Or, the boy may ejaculate during a wet dream.

Wet Dreams

A wet dream is an ejaculation that happens during sleep. Doctors call them *nocturnal emissions*.

Grown men have wet dreams, but they are much more common among boys going through puberty. Not all boys have wet dreams at this time in their lives, but many do. A boy who masturbates regularly may have fewer wet dreams than one who never or only rarely masturbates.

Some boys have their first ejaculation during a wet dream. If you don't know what to expect, a wet dream can be a confusing experience. Some boys think they have wet their beds or are bleeding until they see that the milky white fluid is not like blood or urine. One older man we interviewed described his confusion about wet dreams.

> I'm . . . sixty-seven years old, so this is over fifty years ago, but I still remember my first wet dream like it was yesterday. Nobody told me anything about anything. So I woke up in the middle of the night. There's this wet, sticky stuff all over my belly. I thought, jeez, I wet my bed—at my age! I was thirteen or fourteen at the time.
>
> So a few days, maybe a week later, it happens again. Only now I pay more attention, and it's not piss. It's white and thick like a lotion or cream, sticky. I think I've got some kind of sickness. It keeps happening, so finally I tell my mother. She says if I control myself and don't think about "such things," it won't happen. I have no idea what she's talking

nocturnal emissions (nok-TUR-nuhl) (ee-MIH-shuns)

about—control myself from what? Don't think about what things? I wasn't thinking about anything. I was asleep.

Charlie, age 67

Charlie's mother was wrong. A boy can't stop himself from having wet dreams. They're just something that happens. They're completely natural and normal, and, like masturbation, are part of your body's way of making room for new sperm. Even if you know about wet dreams beforehand, they can be a surprising experience. One boy told me after class:

> My mom and dad had told me all about this kind of stuff ever since I was a kid. Still, it was a surprise the first time. Everything was hazy, but there was this wetness on my pajamas, and for a while I couldn't figure things out. I was only half awake. Then as I woke up more, I thought, "Oh, yeah, this is what Mom had said about."
>
> *Gordon, age 14*

Many boys feel embarrassed when they have a wet dream. One of the films I use in my sex-education classes is called *Am I Normal?* It deals with one boy's experience as he goes through puberty. In one scene, the boy wakes up after having a wet dream. He's so embarrassed that he takes off his pajamas and the sheets off his bed and sneaks down the hall to the bathroom. He turns the water on in the sink and pours a glass of water over his bedclothes and stuffs them in the laundry hamper. His mom hears him and calls out, "Is that you, honey? Is there anything wrong?"

"Nothing, Mom . . . Oh, by the way, Mom, I forgot to tell you . . . I spilled water all over my bed," he nervously explains. "I guess I'm going to have to put my sheets in the hamper."

The boys in my class always get a big laugh out of this scene—probably because many of them have felt the same way. But wet dreams aren't anything to be embarrassed about. They're a natural and normal thing, just another part of growing up.

After I show this film, there are usually questions about wet dreams in the question box. Kids want to know if wet dreams only happen at night. I explain that wet dreams can happen anytime you're asleep. If you take a nap during the day, it's possible for you to have a wet dream. But wet dreams only happen when you're asleep. You won't ejaculate when you're awake, unless you deliberately engage in some form of sexual stimulation.

The kids in my class also want to know if wet dreams only happen during a dream. "Do you have to be having a sexy dream?" they ask. The fact of the matter is that everyone dreams when he or she is asleep. Even if you don't remember any in the morning, you have had dreams during the night. The term wet dream doesn't mean that you always dream. It just refers to the fact that wet dreams happen when you're asleep. You may, or may not, have a "sexy dream." Sometimes, you may awake after a wet dream and recall a sexual dream, but you may have a wet dream without having a sexual dream. It happens both ways.

In this chapter we've talked about a number of topics that interest most boys. We hope the next chapter, that talks about girls and puberty, will prove equally interesting.

CHAPTER 8

Girls and Puberty

As we go through puberty, we usually get some information about what's happening to our own bodies. It comes from our parents, our teachers, and our friends. A lot of times, though, parents and teachers don't tell us about the opposite sex. (They may think that knowing about the opposite sex will make us want to rush out and have sex.) Other boys may not know any more about this subject than you do. However, that doesn't always stop them from spreading a lot of misinformation.

But not knowing what happens in the opposite sex can make puberty more confusing than it needs to be. That's why, in this chapter, we talk about puberty changes in girls' bodies. If you're like most boys, you are probably pretty curious about this. (In fact, we wouldn't be surprised if this is the first chapter you read.)

SIMILARITIES AND DIFFERENCES

As you can see in Figure 40, girls change quite a bit as they go through puberty. In many ways, puberty in girls is similar to puberty in boys. Both sexes undergo a growth spurt and develop more adult body shapes. Both

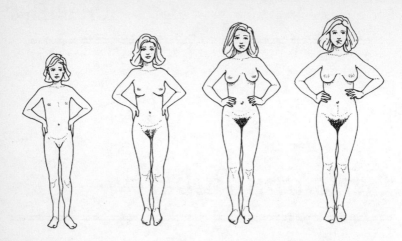

Figure 40. Puberty in Girls. As girls go through puberty, they get taller. Fat tissue begins to grow around their hips, thighs, and buttocks, giving their bodies a curvier shape. Their breasts develop, and they begin to grow pubic hair, as well as hair on their underarms.

boys and girls begin to grow pubic hair. The genital organs of both sexes develop. Boys start to make sperm for the first time, and girls produce their first ripe ovum. Boys and girls begin to perspire more and are likely to get pimples at this time in their lives.

But boys and girls are different. Some changes that happen to boys don't happen to girls. For instance, girls don't experience the same lowering and deepening of the voice that boys do. Also, there are changes that happen to girls that don't happen to boys. For example, boys don't have menstrual periods. The timing of puberty is also different in girls than it is in boys. Puberty usually starts earlier for girls. The average girl starts to develop breasts before the average boy's testicles and penis start to develop. She also begins to grow pubic hair before the average boy. Still, as we know, not everyone is average.

Some girls start later than average. Boys who are early starters may enter puberty before many girls of their age.

Even though boys and girls don't go through all the same changes, their feelings and emotional reactions to growing up are very similar.

THE FIRST CHANGES

For most girls, the first sign of puberty is breast development or the growth of pubic hair (or both). For a smaller number of girls, underarm hair is the first sign of puberty. These changes happen at a wide range of ages. A girl may start puberty when she's only seven or eight. Or, she may not begin pubic hair or breast development until she's thirteen or even older. On the average, girls start puberty between the ages of eight and a half and eleven.

BREASTS

Figure 41 shows the inside of a grown woman's breast. As you can see, a woman's breast contains milk glands and ducts. There is also a good deal of fat to cushion the milk glands. After a woman gives birth, her milk glands begin to produce milk. When a woman breast-feeds, the baby sucks on the nipple. Milk travels through the ducts to the nipple. There are twenty or so tiny openings in the nipple. When the baby sucks, the milk comes out of these openings.

During puberty, a girl's breasts begin to develop. Milk glands and duct tissue develop under each nipple. But her breasts are still not yet ready to make milk. That doesn't happen until she gives birth, and her body is getting ready to nourish a child.

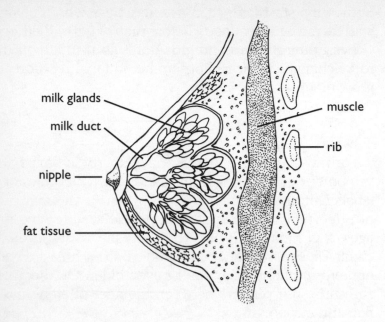

Figure 41. Inside the Breast

Feelings About Developing Breasts

Boys worry about the size of their penises. Girls worry about the size of their breasts. Many girls (and women, too) wish their breasts were larger. As you know, the size of a man's penis has nothing to do with how masculine he is. Likewise the size of a female's breasts has nothing to do with how feminine she is. Breasts work equally well and produce the same amount of milk regardless of their size.

Bras

Once their breasts start developing, many girls begin to wear a bra. Some wear them for support. They feel more comfortable if their breasts don't jiggle around when they run or dance or play sports. Some girls wear bras because they feel self-conscious without them. Other girls may choose not to wear bras at all. It's a matter of personal choice.

THE STAGES OF PUBERTY

Do you recall the five stages of genital development we talked about in Chapter 2? Well, doctors must be fond of fives. They've also divided breast development into five stages. You can see these stages in Figure 42.

Stage 1 is the childhood stage. The breasts have not yet begun to develop. Stage 2 is the beginning of breast development. A small, button-like breast bud forms under each nipple, making the nipple stick out from the chest. The nipple gets larger, and the areola gets wider. Both the nipple and areola darken in color. The breast buds may be tender or even painful. Girls typically reach Stage 2 between the ages of eight and a half and eleven.

In Stage 3, the breasts continue to get larger, rounder, and fuller. They stand out from the chest more. Most girls reach Stage 3 when they are ten to thirteen years old. In Stage 4, the nipple and areola form a separate mound atop the breast. The breasts tend to be rather pointy in this stage. Some girls skip this stage. Typically, girls reach Stage 4 when they are twelve to fourteen. Stage 5 is the adult stage. Usually, girls reach Stage 5 somewhere between thirteen and sixteen years of age. Of course, not all girls are the same. Some girls will reach these stages when they're a bit younger, and some when they're a bit older.

Girls grow pubic hair on the vulva during puberty. There are also five stages of pubic hair growth for girls. These stages are shown in Figure 43.

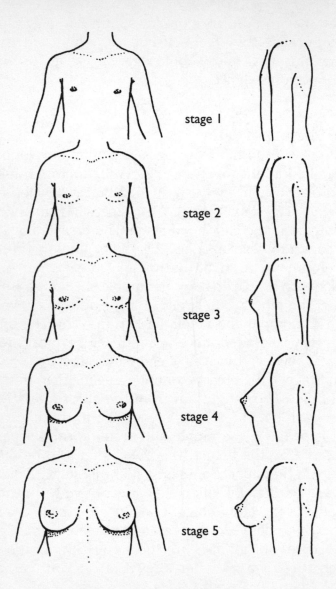

stage 1

stage 2

stage 3

stage 4

stage 5

Figure 42. Five Stages of Breast Development

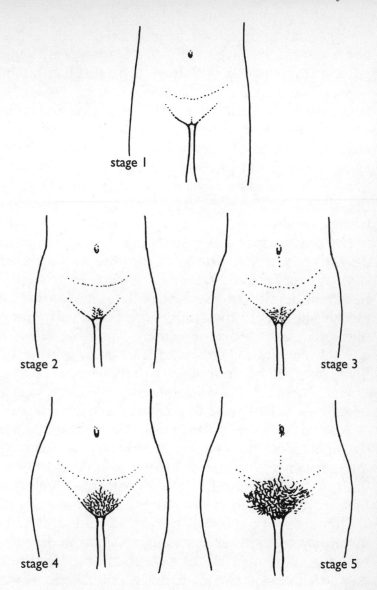

Figure 43. Five Stages of Pubic Hair Growth

Stage 1 is the childhood stage. A girl doesn't have any pubic hair during Stage 1. Stage 2 starts when the first pubic hairs appear. As with boys, these first hairs are not very curly and have little color.

During Stage 3, the pubic hairs get darker and curlier. They cover a wider area and there are more of them, but still not very many. In Stage 4, the pubic hair is as thick and curly as adult pubic hair, but it doesn't cover as much of the vulva as it will in the adult stage. Stage 5 is the adult stage. The pubic hair grows in an upside-down triangle pattern.

The age at which a boy starts puberty has nothing to do with how quickly he goes through its stages. The same is true for girls. When a girl starts to grow pubic hairs and develop breasts has nothing to do with how quickly she gets to the adult stage. Some early starters develop quickly and some slowly. The same is true for late starters and for girls who start at an average age. Some girls will go from Stage 2 to Stage 5 in two years, or less. Other girls take six or more years. The typical girl takes three to four years to go from Stage 2 to Stage 5.

When a boy starts puberty has nothing to do with the size of his penis. Boys who start early don't wind up with a larger penis. The same is true for girls and breasts. Starting early has nothing to do with how big a girl's breasts will be when they mature.

The stages of pubic hair growth and breast development may go together. For example, a girl in Stage 3 of breast development might also be in Stage 3 of pubic hair development. However, this is not always the case. A girl might be in Stage 3 of breast development but only Stage 2 of pubic hair growth. Or, she might be in Stage 3 of pubic hair development and only Stage 2 of breast development.

THE GROWTH SPURT

Like boys, girls go through a growth spurt during puberty. They start to grow taller and heavier at a rapid rate. But unlike boys, girls do not go through a strength spurt.

For girls, the growth spurt happens at the beginning of puberty. For boys, it comes later in puberty. At the age of ten or eleven, girls are often taller than the boys their age. However, after their growth spurt begins a couple of years later, the boys catch up to the girls, and usually end up being taller. Of course, there are some girls who will always be taller than most boys.

Changing Shape

The shape of a girl's body changes as she goes through puberty. Her hips get wider, and fat tissue grows around her hips, buttocks, and thighs. This gives her body a curvier, rounder, more "womanly" shape. As with boys, girls' faces also change and become more adult. However, the change is not as dramatic in girls as it is in boys.

BODY HAIR, PERSPIRATION, PIMPLES, AND OTHER CHANGES

Girls also grow new hair on their arms and legs during puberty. Some girls shave the hair on their legs with razors or remove it with creams, waxes, or some other method. Others don't bother. Again, this is a matter of personal choice.

Like boys, girls develop underarm hair during puberty. Most girls shave this hair. Perspiration and oil glands in the genital area, the underarms, the face, neck, shoulders, and back also become more active in girls. Their body odor changes and they may start using deodorants or antiperspirants. Pimples and acne may be a problem for girls, just as they are for some boys, but, on the whole, girls have less severe acne than boys.

The Sex Organs

A girl's sex organs develop and change during puberty. Figure 2 in Chapter 1 shows the mature sex organs on the outside of a woman's body. It is during puberty that pubic hair grows on the mons and the outer lips of the vulva. The fat pad of the mons gets thicker. The outer and the inner lips get fatter. The outer lips, which are rather flat during childhood, get thicker. The inner lips also develop. Both inner and outer lips get larger, more wrinkly, and darker. The urinary and vaginal openings and the clitoris also get larger.

If you recall from Chapter 1, the tip of the clitoris is partly covered by a hood. This hood is formed by the folds of skin where the inner lips join together. (See Figure 2, page 6.) The rest of the clitoris lies below the surface of the skin. The tip is a small, pink, firm nub of tissue. In a grown woman, it is about the size of the eraser atop a pencil. Like the penis, the clitoris is very sensitive to sexual feelings, thought, and touching.

Masturbation

As you know, boys most often masturbate by touching, rubbing, or stroking the penis in ways that give them sexual pleasure. Girls most often masturbate by touching, rubbing, or stroking the clitoris, or the area around it. As with boys, some girls start to masturbate when they are kids and continue throughout their lives. Others don't masturbate until they start puberty. Some don't start until they are older. And some never masturbate at all. Whether they do or they don't, it's perfectly normal.

Like males, females can have orgasms when they masturbate. In many ways, orgasms are similar in males and females. Both sexes experience a build up of sexual tension and a powerful release of tension during orgasm. However, unlike males, females don't ejaculate when they have an orgasm. The vulva and vagina become moist, or "wet," when a female becomes sexually excited. But this sexual lubrication is not ejaculation.

The Hymen

A girl's *hymen* gets thicker and more noticeable during puberty. The hymen is a thin piece of tissue just inside the vaginal opening. Slang terms for it are "cherry" or "maidenhead."

The hymen looks different in different women. It may be just a thin fringe of skin around the edges of the opening to the vagina. Or, it may stretch across the opening and have one or more holes in it. Figure 44 shows some of the ways a hymen may look.

You may have heard all sorts of stories about the hymen. Many people think that you can tell if a girl is a virgin by the condition of her hymen, but this is not true. (A virgin is a person who has never had sexual intercourse.)

It is true that most hymens are torn or stretched when a woman has sex for the first time. However, some women have sex many times without much stretching or tearing of their hymens. Also, some girls have hymens that look as if they have been stretched or torn even though they haven't been and the girls have never had sex.

hymen (HI-muhn)

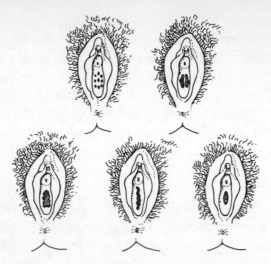

Figure 44. Different Hymens. The hymen may have one or two large openings or several small ones.

When the hymen is stretched or torn, there may or may not bleed be some bleeding. There may be some discomfort, but the pain usually isn't severe or long-lasting.

The Vagina, Uterus, Ovaries, and Uterine Tubes

A girl has sex organs on the inside of her body, too. During puberty these organs also begin to develop and grow (see Figure 45). The vagina gets longer, until it reaches its adult length of three to five inches. This still isn't very large. As you may recall, the average penis is about six inches long when it's erect. However, the vagina is very elastic and stretchy. So, the penis can fit inside when a man and a woman are having sexual intercourse.

The uterus and its tubes get larger during puberty. In a grown woman the uterus is about the size of a fist.

It, too, is very elastic—so much so that it can expand to hold a growing baby.

The ovaries, two small organs on either side of the uterus, also grow larger during puberty. Besides growing, they undergo an even more dramatic change during puberty. They begin producing ripe ova. When a ripe ovum unites with a mature sperm, a baby can grow.

Ovulation

All during your adult life, you will make new sperm. Girls are different. They are born with all the ova they will ever have, but their ova are not fully mature. During puberty they begin to ripen. Sometime after a girl starts puberty, she will ovulate—release a ripe ovum from the ovary—for the first time. Grown women ovulate about once a month. Girls may not ovulate that often at first.

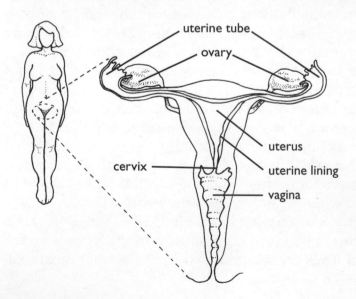

Figure 45. Internal Female Organs

It may take two or three years before they begin to ovulate regularly. A grown woman usually releases a ripe ovum from her ovary about once a month.

Before the ovum even leaves the ovary, the uterus begins preparing for a possible pregnancy. It grows a thick lining where the ovum can plant itself if it is fertilized. New blood vessels develop in the lining which can carry blood to an implanted ovum. The lining also begins to secrete nutrients to nourish the ovum in the early stages of pregnancy.

MENSTRUATION

Most of the time, the ovum doesn't get fertilized by a sperm. Therefore, it doesn't plant itself in the uterine lining. Instead, it simply dissolves soon after it arrives in the uterus.

Since the ovum isn't fertilized, the newly grown lining is not needed. About a week after the ovum dissolves, the uterus begins to shed the lining. Pieces of the lining slide off the walls of the uterus. The spongy, blood-filled tissue breaks down, becoming mostly liquid. This liquid is called *menstrual* blood or the menstrual flow. It collects in the bottom of the uterus. From there, it dribbles into the vagina and out the vaginal opening (see Figure 46).

It may take anywhere from three to seven days for the uterus to shed its lining. On the average, the menstrual flow lasts for five days. During this time, a girl is said to be *menstruating*, or having her menstrual period.

While she's having her period, a girl usually wears a menstrual pad or a tampon to prevent leakage of the blood. Pads are made of layers of absorbent material,

menstrual (MEN-stroo-uhl)
menstruating (MEN-stroo-ay-ting)

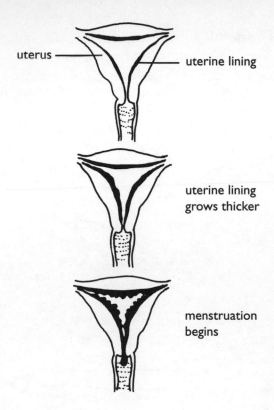

uterus ——— uterine lining

uterine lining
grows thicker

menstruation
begins

Figure 46. Menstruation. As the ovary gets ready to release a ripe ovum, the uterine lining grows thicker. If the ovum is not fertilized the uterine lining breaks down and is shed causing menstruation to begin.

which are worn inside the underpants. Tampons are absorbent cotton plugs, which are inserted into the vagina (see Figure 47).

A girl generally has her first menstrual period sometime between the ages of nine and sixteen. The average age is twelve or thirteen. Some girls are excited about the prospect of having their periods; others aren't so

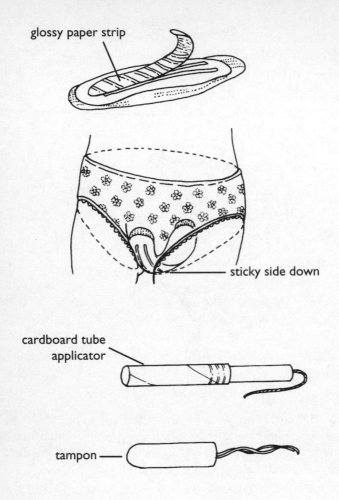

glossy paper strip

sticky side down

cardboard tube applicator

tampon

Figure 47. Menstrual Protection. Most girls use either pads or tampons to absorb menstrual flow. The pad shown in this Figure has an adhesive side that is covered with a glossy strip of paper. When that strip of paper is pulled off, the pad is held sticky side down inside the panties. Tampons are absorbent plugs that are inserted into the vagina. They usually come inside a cardboard or plastic applicator.

eager. Many girls are concerned that their first period will sneak up on them. They worry that the blood will soak through their clothes without their knowing it and they'll be embarrassed. Such things can happen, but usually a girl senses the wetness and has time to get to the bathroom. Besides, not that much blood comes out all at once. Altogether over the entire period, only about a quarter to a third of a cup of blood is lost. So, only a small amount is dribbling out of the vaginal opening at any one time.

The Menstrual Cycle

After the uterus has shed its lining, the menstrual period stops. Meanwhile, another ovum is already ripening for ovulation. Soon after the menstrual bleeding stops, the uterine lining starts to grow thick again, getting ready for the next ovulation and another possibility of pregnancy.

In a grown woman, ovulation happens about once a month. (It's once every twenty-eight days on the average.) About a month after the previous ovulation, the ovary releases another ripe ovum. It travels through the uterine tube toward the uterus. If the ovum is not fertilized, the newly grown lining will again be shed and another menstrual period will begin.

This cycle of menstruation and ovulation is called the menstrual cycle (see Figure 48). The whole cycle runs from the first day of bleeding during one period to the first day of bleeding of the next period. On the average, one cycle takes twenty-eight days, but, few women have their periods every twenty-eight days like clockwork. The length of the cycle may vary from one cycle to the next and also from one woman to the next. Young

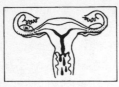

Days 1-5: During the first five days, the uterine lining is being shed and the girl is having her period. At the same time ova begin to mature.

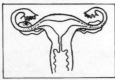

Days 6-13: During these days, ova continue maturing. Also, the uterine lining begins to grow thick and rich in nutrients.

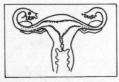

Day 14: On day 14 of the typical twenty-eight day cycle, ovulation occurs. Usually only one ovum is released.

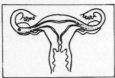

Days 14-19: During these days, the ovum travels through the uterine tube toward the uterus. The uterine lining continues to thicken.

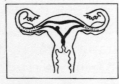

Day 20: The ovum reaches the uterus on about day 20 of the typical cycle.

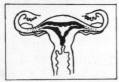

Days 21-28: If it hasn't been fertilized, the ovum will dissolve, and the uterine lining will be shed. Bleeding will begin again on the 29th day, which is day 1 of the next cycle.

Figure 48. Menstrual Cycle. A typical menstrual cycle lasts twenty-eight days. However, the length of a menstrual cycle may be quite a bit longer or shorter than twenty-eight days. Young girls, who have just started menstruating, are especially likely to have longer, and irregular menstrual cycles.

women are especially likely to have irregular cycles. It takes two or three years to establish regular cycles. Some girls never do get very regular.

The menstrual cycle repeats itself over and over for much of a woman's adult life. The cycle stops while a woman is pregnant. Illness, stress, and breastfeeding can also cause a woman miss to periods. But, by and large, except for when she is pregnant, a woman continues to menstruate and ovulate until she reaches *menopause*.

Puberty is the time in a girl's life when menstrual periods begin. Menopause is the time in a woman's life when they stop.

It usually happens when a woman is between the ages of forty-five and fifty-five.

Hormones

As you may recall from Chapter 6, puberty begins in the brain. In both boys and girls, chemicals made in the brain travel to the pituitary gland. There, they cause the pituitary to start making hormones.

In boys, the pituitary hormones travel to the testicles. They cause the testicles to make the hormone testosterone. In girls, the pituitary hormones travel to the ovaries. They cause the ovaries to make the hormone *estrogen*.

In boys, testosterone helps the testicles produce sperm. It also causes the enlargement of the testicles and penis, lowered voice, muscle development, and other puberty changes. In girls, estrogen helps the ova to ripen in the ovary. It also causes the sex organs to

menopause (MEN-o-paws)
estrogen (ES-tro-jen)

mature, the breasts to develop, and other puberty changes to occur.

Estrogen also helps to control the menstrual cycle. In the first half of the menstrual cycle, before ovulation, the ovaries make increasing amounts of estrogen. The estrogen helps the ova to ripen. After ovulation, the ovaries begin to make another hormone called *progesterone*. The levels of these two hormones from the ovary rise and fall over the course of the menstrual cycle and control the process of menstruation and ovulation.

Menstrual Cramps

Menstrual cramps are abdominal pains that sometimes accompany the menstrual flow. They usually begin as the bleeding starts or shortly before. They usually last for one to three days. They vary from a feeling of heaviness, to a dull ache, to sharp, cramp-like pain. They're usually worse in the first twenty-four to thirty-six hours.

Almost every woman has cramps at some time in her life, but for most, they're not a real problem and don't interfere with daily activities. However, some have severe cramps and actually have to spend a few days in bed.

Cramps are more common in teenagers than in older women. Nowadays, doctors have effective treatments that usually work, even on severe cramps. There are also effective treatments for cramps that can be purchased without a doctor's prescription.

Other Menstrual Changes and PMS

Some girls and women notice changes in their bodies or in their emotions that begin during certain times in their menstrual cycles. These changes might be pleasant

progesterone (pro-JES-ter-own)

ones like extra energy, an especially good feeling, or a burst of creativity. Or they might be negative changes like tension, headaches, bowel problems, swelling, or temporary weight gain. Some girls notice that they're cranky right before their period starts. Or they are more apt to get depressed at this time.

Girls who have negative changes before their menstrual period may have premenstrual syndrome, or PMS. No one is sure what causes PMS. Some doctors think that vitamin and nutritional deficiencies cause it. Others think that it's a hormone imbalance. Most women have some symptoms.

I hope this chapter has helped you learn something about puberty changes in girls. Remember, the more information you have, the less confusing puberty is.

CHAPTER 9

Romantic and Sexual Feelings

I think I might be sex-crazy or something. I mean, I'm always thinking about girls, fantasizing, and I masturbate a lot, like at least twice a day. Do you think I'm okay?

Anonymous, Question Box

Questions like this come up a lot because, as we go through puberty, many of us experience strong romantic and/or sexual feelings. For some boys, this means spending time imagining a passionate romance with a special someone or having sexual fantasies. For some boys, it means having the urge to masturbate more often. For some, it means getting interested in the opposite sex, having crushes, or having a romance.

These romantic and sexual feelings can be very strong. At times, it may even seem as if romance and sex are all you can think about! Some young people get so wrapped up that it's a bit scary for them. If you sometimes worry about how intense your romantic or sexual feelings are, it helps to know that these feelings are perfectly normal. A lot of people your age are going through the same thing.

But not everyone experiences such strong sexual or romantic feelings during puberty. Some boys are more involved in sports, school, music, or whatever. So sometimes we get questions like this:

> My friends are always talking about sex and everything. I'm just not interested in the romance thing. Do you think there's something wrong with me?
>
> *Anonymous, Question Box*

Just as we each have our own timetable of development when it comes to the body changes of puberty, we also have our own timetable for romance and sexual interests. So there's no need to worry because everyone else your age is all wrapped up in sex and you're not. There's nothing wrong with you. Your personal timetable is just different from theirs. You have lots of time ahead of you to experience your sexual and romantic feelings.

The boys in my classes are curious about anything and everything having to do with sex. And they're especially curious about the kinds of romantic and sexual feelings that young people have when they're growing up. We talked about fantasies and masturbation earlier in this book. But having fantasies and masturbating are usually private things that you do by yourself. In this chapter, we'll be talking more about your sexual and romantic feelings that involve other people. We'll be talking about things like crushes, dating and falling in love. But first, we'd like to say a couple of things about friendships.

"JUST FRIENDS"

When we're small children no one makes much of a fuss over the fact that two kids of the opposite sex are friends. Once in a while, people will make cracks about "puppy love." But it's just not a big deal if a little boy and girl play together, are best friends, or spend the night at each others' houses. As puberty approaches, though, things change. Suddenly, it's no longer okay to spend the night at your best friend's house if your best friend happens to be someone of the opposite sex. The other kids at school or the adults around suddenly start assuming that you must be more than "just friends." They assume you like each other in a romantic, boyfriend/girlfriend sort of way.

At least, the kids in my classes often say that it's harder to be "just friends" after you reach a certain age. Here's what one girl in my class had to say:

> I'm going to Paul's Halloween party on Saturday, and my brother keeps teasing me, "Oh, you like Paul, you're in love with Paul." Well, I do like Paul, but not like that. All of a sudden, you can't just be friends with a boy. It's got to be boyfriend or girlfriend, like you're all romantic with each other.
>
> *Felicia, age 13*

An eleven-year-old boy had been friends with a girl since they were little kids. He had this to say:

> I went over to Hilary's house to spend the night, and we were swimming in the pool. These girls who live next door came over and they were saying things like, "Oh, you're playing with a girl. Oh, you're staying overnight at a girl's house. Oh, that's weird."
>
> *Donny, age 11*

Many kids complain about this sort of teasing and how people just assume that a friend of the opposite sex is more than "just a friend." So, in class, we talk about how to handle this problem. Here's some advice we've come up with:

- Just ignore the teasing and rumors. Take a "so what" attitude. After all, who cares if they think you're madly in love with your friend?
- Explain to people that you are "just friends." Tell them why you think it's fun or a good idea or whatever to be "just friends."
- Talk to your friend about it so the teasing or rumors don't make you feel uncomfortable around each other.

If you're having problems in this way, try some of this advice. Don't let "the romance thing" keep you from enjoying an opposite-sex friendship.

CRUSHES

Of course, sometimes we are interested in romance. In fact, many boys develop crushes. Having a crush means having romantic or sexual feelings towards a certain, special someone. Crushes can be very exciting. Just thinking about or catching a glimpse of the person you have a crush on can brighten your whole day. You may spend delightful hours imagining a romance with that special someone.

Sometimes boys develop crushes on someone who isn't very likely to return their affections. It might be a film star, a rock singer, a teacher, another adult, or a friend of an older brother or sister. These sorts of crushes can be a safe and healthy way of experimenting with romantic and sexual feelings. Still, no matter how much we may pretend otherwise, deep down we know that this person is unattainable. So, we don't have to worry about real-life problems like what to say or how to act. We're free to imagine what we like, without worrying about whether that person will be attracted to us. In a way, having a crush on an "unattainable someone" is a way of rehearsing for the time when we will have a real-life romance.

But having this kind of crush can also be painful. If you find yourself developing a serious crush on someone unattainable, it helps to remind yourself from time to time that your crush isn't very realistic. This person isn't very likely to return your affections.

Not all crushes are unrealistic. You may develop a crush on someone near your own age whom you actually know through school, church, temple, or whatever. If that person shows an interest in you as well, the crush can be especially exciting, but yearning after a person who doesn't return your affections can hurt. If your crushes are causing you problems, it helps to discuss your feelings with someone. That person might be a friend, a parent, a teacher, another adult, or a counselor.

When boys talk with us about being romantically or sexually interested in someone they actually know, they often ask: *How do you find out if someone likes you? How do you let someone know how you feel?*

There are basically two ways: You can do it on your own, or you can have a friend do it for you.

If you decide to have a friend do it, you'll want to pick someone you really trust. You don't want it known all over school! It's often easier to let someone else do the talking for you. But keep in mind that if you do this, you don't have very much control over what's being said. Suppose, for example, you only want your friend to bring up your name in a roundabout way and see how this other person reacts. Instead, your friend might make it sound as if you're madly in love with this person you're interested in!

For these reasons, many people prefer to do it on their own. There are a lot of ways to let someone know how you feel. You can be friendly, start conversations, go out of your way to be around that person, ask the person to go out with you, or simply tell the person how you feel. You can also watch to see if that person does any of these sorts of things to *you*. If so, chances are that person likes you.

Regardless of whether you tell the person yourself or have a friend do it for you, make sure it's done in private. It may embarrass the person to talk about feelings for you in front of friends or classmates. As a result, the person might really like you but not want to say so in front of everyone.

HOMOSEXUAL FEELINGS

Sometimes people have crushes on people of the same sex. When we talk about this in class it always brings up questions about *homosexuality*.

Homo means "same." Having homosexual feelings means having romantic or sexual feelings, fantasies, dreams, or crushes about someone of the same sex. Many boys and girls have homosexual thoughts or feelings or actual sexual experiences with someone of the same sex, while they're growing up.

If you've had homosexual feelings or experiences, you may know that this is quite normal. You may not be at all worried about it. Or, you may feel somewhat confused or upset, or even downright scared, by these kinds of feelings or experiences. Perhaps you've heard people making jokes or using insulting slang terms when talk-

homosexuality (ho-mo-SEK-shoo-AL-eh-tee)

ing about homosexuality. If so, this may have caused you to wonder if your homosexual feelings or experiences are really okay. Perhaps you have heard someone say that homosexuality is morally wrong, sinful, abnormal, or a sign of mental sickness. If so, this, too, may have made you worry about your own feelings. If you've heard any of these things (or even if you haven't), we think it will be helpful for you to know the basic facts about homosexuality.

Almost everyone has homosexual thoughts, feelings, fantasies, or experiences at some time or another in their lives. That's why we usually consider people to be homosexuals only if, as adults, their strongest romantic and sexual attractions are toward someone of the same sex. Usually most of their actual sexual experiences will also involve someone of the same sex. About one in every ten adults in our society is a homosexual.

Both males and females can be homosexuals. Female homosexuals are called *lesbians.* "Gay" is a noninsulting slang term for either male or female homosexuals. There have been homosexuals throughout history, including some very famous people. People from any social class, ethnic background, religious affiliation, or economic level may be homosexual. Doctors, nurses, lawyers, bus drivers, police officers, artists, business people, ministers, rabbis, priests, teachers, politicians, football players, married people, single people, parents—you name it— all sorts of people are homosexuals.

The majority of adults in our society are heterosexual people. *Hetero* means "opposite." Heterosexuals have strong romantic and sexual attractions toward the oppo-

lesbian (LES-bee-uhn)

site sex. Most of their actual sexual experiences involve the opposite sex.

We've talked about a few basic facts, but if you're like most of the boys in my classes you probably still have questions about homosexuality. Here are answers to a few of their questions.

Is homosexuality morally wrong? Is it unnatural, abnormal, or a sign of a mental sickness?

In the past, many people felt that homosexuality was sinful or abnormal. There are still some people who feel this way. However, nowadays, more and more people no longer believe this. We feel that it's a personal matter, that some people happen to be homosexuals and that being homosexual is a perfectly healthy, normal, and acceptable way to be.

What's a bisexual?

A *bisexual* is a person who is equally attracted to males and females and whose sexual activities may involve either sex.

If a person has a lot of homosexual feelings or fools around with someone of the same sex while growing up, will this person be a homosexual as an adult?

Having homosexual feelings and experiences while you're growing up doesn't mean you'll be a homosexual as an adult. Many of the young people who have homosexual feelings and experiences while they're growing up turn out to be heterosexuals as adults. And quite naturally, some turn out to be homosexuals.

bisexual (bye-SEK-shoo-uhl)

We've talked to many adults who are homosexuals about their feelings when they were growing up, and have gotten many different answers. Some had homosexual feelings while they were growing up. Others had heterosexual feelings. Still others didn't have strong sexual feelings one way or the other as they were growing up.

Can a person know for sure that they're gay even though they're still young?
Yes. At least, some gay adults say that they knew they were homosexuals when they were teenagers. Some even say they knew when they were small children.

For more information about homosexuality, you can consult the resources listed on pages 228–229.

DATING
As young people move through puberty and into their teen years, many begin dating. This can be fun and exciting, but it can also create problems. For instance, you may want to date before your parents think you're old enough. Or you may not feel ready to date, and your parents or friends may be pushing you into it. You may have trouble deciding whether you want to go steady with one person or go out with different people. If you've been dating one person regularly and decide you want to date others, it may be hard to end your steady dating relationship. Or, if your "steady" wants to change the relationship, you may get hurt and have a hard time coping. On the other hand, you may want to date and no one is interested in going out with you. This could make you feel rather depressed.

Here again, if you're having dating problems, it might be helpful to talk them over with someone you respect and trust. You might talk to one of your parents, another adult you trust, a friend, or an older brother or sister. In addition, it might be helpful for you to hear some of the questions that come up in my classes about this topic.

Suppose that you'd like to date, but you never have and you're beginning to wonder if you ever will?

If the other kids you know have already started dating, but you haven't, you may get to feeling that you won't ever start. If so, it helps to remember that we each have our own timetable when it comes to romantic matters, too. It can seem awfully hard if your personal timetable is moving along more slowly than other people's, but the fact that you're getting a slow start doesn't mean that you won't ever start dating. It may take a while, but eventually, you'll start dating, too. We guarantee it!

Remember, you've got many years ahead of you. It doesn't really matter if you start dating when you're only thirteen years old or not until you're twenty. What's important in the long run is that you feel good about yourself.

What if every time you ask someone out, the answer is "no"?

If you've asked a person out a number of times and the person keeps saying "no," you may just have to face the fact that this person doesn't want to go out with you. It can be difficult to know exactly how many times you should ask before giving up altogether. Partly, it will depend on what the person says. If you're told that the person is already dating someone else or simply isn't interested in you, that's pretty clear. You should stop asking. But, if you're told, "I'm sorry, but I'm busy," you might want to try again. Perhaps the person would like to go out but really is busy. If you keep trying and get this kind of reply each time, you might want to say something like, "I'd love to hear from you if you ever have some time free," and leave it at that. The person can then choose to follow up on that invitation—or not.

If you've asked a number of different people out and all of them have said "no," you may begin feeling awfully discouraged. You may even start to feel that something is so wrong or so horrible about you that no one will ever say "yes." Before you allow yourself to feel down and discouraged, think for a moment. Who are you asking out? Maybe they're the wrong people! Are you only asking the best-looking or most popular people? If so, this may be part of your problem. For one thing, the best-looking and most popular people may already have lots of other people asking them out. Your chances might be better if you asked someone less popular or not-totally-gorgeous. Besides, the fact that someone is popular or good-looking doesn't necessarily mean you're going to have a great time on a date. What's more important is whether the person is nice. Can the two of you be comfortable with each other? Can you have fun together? A person's inner qualities are a lot more important than being popular or good-looking.

You might also ask yourself how well you know the person you're asking out. If you're asking someone you hardly know, this may be a big part of the reason you keep getting turned down. Take the time to get to know someone and let that person get to know you first. Then you're more likely to get a "yes" answer when you ask for a date.

It might also be helpful for you to have a mutual friend check things out before you ask for a date. Your friend can give you an idea of how the person might respond. If there's no interest, you'll save yourself the discouragement of being turned down. In addition, you might ask some of your friends who *they* think you should ask for a date. People love to play matchmaker. Your friends may come up with someone you wouldn't have thought of on your own. They may even know someone who's been dying to go out with you! So don't hesitate to ask for your friends' help.

Suppose you want to date, but your parents say "no"?

Young people usually choose to handle this problem in one of three ways: (1) sneak around behind their parents' backs; (2) go along with their parents' rules and wait until their parents say they're old enough; or (3) try and change their parents' minds. Let's look at each of these choices.

Sneaking around just isn't a good idea. If you get caught, you may get into a lot of trouble. Also, your parents may find it hard to trust you in the future. Even if you don't get caught, you'll probably feel awfully guilty about lying. And feeling guilty isn't much fun. In the end sneaking around really isn't worth the price you have to pay.

On the other hand, it can be awfully hard to just go along with your parents' rules and wait until you're older. It's especially hard if there's a special someone you'd like to date. But parents usually aren't trying to be mean or unfair. They're trying to protect you from "getting in over your head" by dating at too young an age. Maybe they're right. If your parents say "no," ask yourself these questions: Are most of the other kids my age allowed to date? Would I really lose anything by waiting until I'm older?

If your honest answer to these two questions is "no," then perhaps waiting is the best choice for you. However, you may feel that your parents are being too strict or too old-fashioned. In that case, you might want to consider the third choice, changing their minds.

This may not be easy, but it's worth a try. For starters, find out exactly why they've made these rules. What are they worried about? Once you hear them out, you may be able to come up with a compromise. If, for instance, your parents think you're too young to go out on a solo date, maybe they'd allow you to go on group dates. Or, if they won't allow dates for the movies, perhaps they'll allow you to go to a boy–girl party or invite someone to your house.

FALLING IN LOVE

Many young people fall in love, or at least what they think might be love, but, how do you know when it's really love?

Emotions can't be weighed or measured and different people have different ideas of what it means to be in love, so we can't tell you exactly what real love is. We can, however, share with you some of our thoughts on the subject.

We think it's important to recognize the differences between *infatuation* and true love. Infatuation is an intense, exciting (and sometimes confusing or scary) fireworks kind of feeling. You may be so wrapped up in your infatuation that it's hard to think about anything else.

infatuation (in-FACH-u-a-shun)

People sometimes mistake infatuation for love, especially because they may both start out the same way, but they're not the same. Infatuation usually doesn't last very long. True love does. In addition, you don't have to know someone very well in order to be infatuated, but in order to truly love someone, you have to know that person (both their good qualities and bad ones) very well. Infatuation can happen all of a sudden. True love takes more time. You may start out being infatuated and have it grow into true love. Or, the infatuation may pass and you may discover that you aren't really "right" for each other, after all.

Your relationship may start with the fireworks of an infatuation, or it may develop more slowly and gradually. In either case, a love relationship will sooner or later go through a questioning stage. One or both of you will question whether this relationship is really a good one. During this questioning stage, one of you may decide to end the relationship. In our opinion, it's only after you go through this questioning stage and decide to stay together that you're really on the road to true love.

MAKING DECISIONS ABOUT HOW TO HANDLE YOUR ROMANTIC AND SEXUAL FEELINGS

Young people often face questions about how to handle their strong romantic and sexual feelings. When two people are attracted to each other, they quite naturally want to be physically close. Being physically close may mean something as simple as holding hands or kissing good night after a date. Or, it may mean more than this. Physical closeness may even include something as intimate as sexual intercourse.

Some young people answer questions about how to handle their sexual and romantic feelings based on what they think "everyone else" is doing. Often they're wrong about what "everyone else" is doing. Besides, *just because "everyone else" does it, does not mean it's right for you.*

Other young people just "go along" with what their parents or their religions say is right or wrong, without really thinking much about it. Now, please don't misunderstand what we're saying here. We're not saying that you shouldn't follow your parents' or your religion's teachings or rules. In fact, we think parents and religions have excellent advice that's well worth following. But we've found that young people who accept, without question, what they've been taught sometimes run into problems. When they're actually in romantic situations, they often aren't able to stick to the rules they've been taught. The rules sort of "fall apart" or "cave in" in the face of tremendous pressure to experiment sexually. We think this sometimes happens because the rules weren't really "theirs" in the first place.

A lot of young people, maybe most of them, aren't at all sure what's right or wrong. They look for answers when it comes to deciding how far to go.

If there were one set of answers that everyone agreed with, it would be easy. We could just tell you the answers, but it's not that simple. Different people have different ideas on these issues. So, in class—especially in the classes for older boys and girls—we usually spend a good deal of time on this topic. We discuss making decisions about how to handle romantic and sexual feelings. We explain why people feel the way they do, without "taking sides" one way or the other.

Not until you give it some thought and decide for yourself what rules to follow will the rules become truly your own. And it's not until the rules are truly your own that they become rules you can live by.

When it comes to making decisions about sex, there are many things to consider. There isn't enough space here to cover everything you might need to know. For example, you can't make responsible decisions to have sexual intercourse without being well informed about birth control and sexually transmitted diseases. (See the boxes on pages 204–205 and 207.) But, before we leave this topic, we'd like to answer a couple of questions that often come up in our classes.

I'd like to have a girlfriend, but is someone my age (eleven) old enough to have sex?

I'm twelve and there's a certain boy in my class that I like, and he likes me, too. I'm scared of having sex, though. What should I do?

It's usually younger boys and girls who ask these sorts of questions. When I first heard questions like these, I was a bit shocked that boys and girls who were so young seemed to be asking questions about whether they were ready for sex.

However, in talking further with the young kids who asked these sorts of questions, I understood why they were asking these questions. It was because they often had very mistaken ideas about physical closeness. Some of them thought that kissing or being physically close in other ways happens as soon as you get involved with someone. Some thought that going on a date means you have to, at the very least, kiss the person good night or perhaps even go further. Some even thought that having a boyfriend or girlfriend automatically means that you're going to have sexual intercourse with that person.

These things just aren't true, but it's easy to see how kids get these mistaken ideas. In the books we read, it often seems as if two people who meet on one page will be madly kissing each other on the next page. In the movies, it sometimes seems as if two perfect strangers take one look at each other, and the next thing we know they're in bed together!

Please don't be confused by what you read in books or see on TV or in the movies. Dating or having boyfriends doesn't mean that you have to have sex or even kiss. Dating is, after all, a chance to get to know the person you're going out with. Once you know each other better, you may not want to have any kind of romantic or physical relationship. Above all, remember that when it comes to romance and sex, you're in charge. You don't have to do anything that doesn't feel right for you.

Is it all right to kiss on your first date?
Is it wrong to get into necking?
How far is "too far" to go?
Where should a person draw the line?

As we explained earlier, if everyone agreed upon these issues, these would be easy questions to answer. But, of course, they don't. For instance, some people think it's not right to kiss on a first date, while others think it's perfectly okay to do so. Some people think necking is okay. Others don't. Some people think it's "sinful" to go beyond necking. Some don't think this is morally wrong, but are afraid that young people might get "carried away" and wind up going further than they really meant to.

Young people's answers to the sorts of questions listed above are strongly influenced by their personal situations. Their parents' values, their friends' opinions, their religion's teachings, their own moral beliefs, and their own emotional feelings are all important. These influences affect each of us differently, but we think the following guidelines can be helpful to anyone facing these questions:

- Whether it's French-kissing, necking, or going further, don't let yourself be rushed into anything. Do only what you're really sure you want to do. After all, you have many years ahead of you; you can afford to wait until you are sure.
- Ask yourself how you feel about this other person. Is this someone you trust? Will this person start rumors or gossip about you? Are you doing these things because you really care about this person or simply because you're curious to try these things?
- Are you just trying to prove you're grown up, or trying to become more popular?
- Don't pressure someone into doing something he or she doesn't want to do. This pressure may take the form of a boy persuading a girl to go further than she really wants to. But boys are not the only

BIRTH CONTROL

If a male and female want to have sexual intercourse, but don't want a pregnancy, they can use some form of birth control. Some young people believe that you can't get pregnant the first time you have sex. This is *not true*. There are many, many women who have gotten pregnant the first time they had sex. Young people who have been having sex for a while without getting pregnant develop a false sense of confidence.

They figure that since they've gotten away with it so far, they'll continue to get away with it. This is also *not true*. In fact, the longer a couple continues to have sexual intercourse without using birth control, the greater the chances of pregnancy. Some young people think, "It can't happen to me." They think pregnancy only happens to other people. Again, *not true*. Any couple having sex without using birth control may get pregnant, and most of them do sooner or later.

While we're on the subject of things that are not true, it is also not true that you can't get pregnant if you jump up and down after you have sex. This will not "shake the sperm out." It is not true that a female can't get pregnant if she has sex during her menstrual period. It is not true that douching after sex will prevent pregnancy. And it is not true that a woman can't get pregnant if a man pulls his penis out of her vagina before he ejaculates. During an erection, a male produces a few drops of fluid from the end of his penis. This fluid may contain sperm. Even if a man pulls out before ejaculating, he may still leave some sperm in the vagina. Also, if he ejaculates near the opening to the vagina, the sperm may still be able to swim up into the vagina.

Even if you're not having sex yet, it's a good idea to learn about birth control. There are many different methods. The birth control pill is one of the best methods of preventing pregnancy, but it requires a doctor's prescription. Other methods can be purchased at the store without a prescription, but these methods may not be as effective as the pill.

Condoms are made of latex rubber and fit over the penis like a glove fits over a finger. They prevent the man's semen from getting into the vagina during ejaculation. The condom also helps to protect against sexually transmitted diseases. And, you don't need a doctor's prescription to buy condoms.

There are many choices when it comes to birth control. It's important to become well informed so that you can eventually choose what is best for you. To learn more, see the resources listed on pages 224–225.

ones to apply pressure. A girl may act like a boy isn't "manly" if he doesn't want to kiss or doesn't try to get her to go further.

You may still be unsure about your own decisions and how to handle your sexual feelings. That's not surprising. There are so many aspects to consider—emotional, psychological, physical, spiritual, and moral (to mention just a few). It's always a good idea to wait until you're older, giving yourself time to consider all these things before you decide about sex.

In the end, of course, you're the one who decides. But you might find it useful to talk this over with other people.

Don't (as many young people do) automatically rule out your parents as people to talk to. You may be surprised to find that your parents struggled with these same questions when they were your age. Often young people know that their parents' attitudes are more conservative or stricter than theirs. As a result they may not talk about sexual decision-making with their parents. But even if this is so, your parents may have good reasons for feeling the way they do. And even if you don't totally agree with them, they might have things to say that could prove useful to you. You might also talk with an aunt or uncle, a sister or brother, or an older friend.

SEXUALITY: FEELING PRIVATE/FEELING GUILTY

Even though we haven't actually used the word *sexuality*, we've been talking about sexuality throughout this

sexuality (SEK-shoo-ahl-eh-tee)

AIDS AND OTHER STDS

If you decide to have sexual intercourse, you also need to know about sexually transmitted diseases. Sexually transmitted diseases are also called *STDs*, venereal diseases, or VD. They are infections that are usually transmitted from one person to another through sexual contact. There are a number of different kinds of STDs. The most common ones are gonorrhea, syphilis, chlamydia, venereal warts, and herpes. Gonorrhea, chlamydia, and syphilis can be cured, but if they are not treated promptly, they can cause serious illness. There is no cure for herpes or venereal warts. Herpes has caused birth defects in the babies of some infected mothers. Venereal warts can increase the chance of getting certain types of cancer.

AIDS is the most serious of all diseases that can be sexually transmitted. AIDS attacks the body's immune system and cannot be cured. Although it can be controlled to some extent with drugs, AIDS often leads to death.

Because STDs are transmitted through sexual activity, people are often embarrassed to seek treatment or to tell their sex partners that they may have given them an STD. Before you have sex, you need to learn the signs and symptoms of STDs, how to avoid getting an STD, and what to do if you get one. To learn more about STDs, see the resource section, pages 224–225.

chapter. In fact, this whole book is about sexuality. Some people think the word sexuality only applies to sexual intercourse, but it also includes things like your general attitudes about sex, feelings about your changing body, romantic and sexual fantasies, masturbation, childhood sex play, homosexual feelings, crushes, hugging, kissing, necking, and being physically close in other ways.

Feeling Private

Most people feel private, shy, or even a bit embarrassed about some aspect of their sexuality. Some young people, for instance, become very modest during puberty, and no longer feel okay about family members seeing them nude. Some feel embarrassed asking questions or talking about the changes happening in their bodies. Some feel very private about starting their periods or having wet dreams. They may not want their families or friends to know that these things have happened.

Private feelings can also center on romantic and sexual feelings or activities. Some kids are shy about the fact that they have a crush. Others feel embarrassed about their fantasies or about homosexual feelings. For most, masturbation is something that's very private. Young people may also feel shy about things like kissing and necking, and other kinds of physical closeness. Some feel embarrassed even talking about these things, let alone actually doing them.

Some kids even worry about the fact that sexuality is such a private thing for them, but, feeling private, shy, or even a bit embarrassed about sexuality is completely natural. It doesn't mean that you're "hung up" or "uptight" or that there's something wrong with you. It just means that you're normal!

Feeling Guilty

There is, however, a difference between feeling *private* about your sexuality and feeling *guilty* about it. Some kids don't just feel private, shy, or embarrassed. They also feel guilty, ashamed, "dirty," or otherwise bad about some aspect of their sexuality.

When young people tell us they're having these guilty feelings, we suggest that they ask themselves this question. Is what I'm feeling guilty about something that is (or could be) harmful to myself or others? If it's not, then our advice is to try and let go of the guilty feelings. On the other hand, it may be something that is harmful. In that case, our advice is that you stop doing whatever it is that causes the guilty feelings. Also, make amends, if possible, and decide not to do it in the future.

Even when a person *has* done something harmful, it's often something that's not too serious. For instance, you might feel guilty because you've been flirting with your best friend's steady. But this isn't really all that serious. At least, it's not as serious as the kind of situation described by a fifteen-year-old boy. He felt guilty about having pressured his girlfriend to go further than she really wanted to:

> Necking is as far as she'd ever go because of her moral standards. I kept pushing and got her to, well . . . not actual intercourse, but further than she wanted to go. I didn't force her or anything. I was coming on strong, though. Now I feel like some kind of pervert, and I can tell she doesn't feel good about herself. It's changed things between us. We're not so close.
>
> *Edward, age 15*

This boy did something that was harmful to his girlfriend's good feelings about herself and to his own good feelings about himself. It also hurt their relationship.

In other cases, the harm may be even more serious. For example, suppose a pregnancy resulted from rushing into unprotected sexual intercourse. In this case the harm done is quite serious indeed. Generally speaking, the more serious the harm, the harder it is to deal with the guilt. And, even though you've changed your behavior and done what you can to make amends, this doesn't mean your guilt will go away completely.

It's important to remember that human beings are, after all, *human.* We do make mistakes. If you've done what you can to make amends and change your behavior, then try to forgive yourself and get on with your life.

We also want to remind you of the fact that different people have different ideas about what is or isn't harmful. Take, for example, masturbation, which is something many young people feel guilty about. Personally we think masturbating is a perfectly normal and healthy thing to do. Unless it goes against a person's moral principles, we usually advise young people who are feeling guilty about masturbating to try and relax and let go of the guilt. However, some people see things quite differently. They believe that masturbation is sinful or morally wrong and that people do themselves harm in a moral sense by masturbating. Because of these beliefs their advice would probably be just the opposite of ours. They might advise young people to stop masturbating, and not to masturbate again in the future.

How people react to situations where they feel guilty depends not only on how serious any harm done may be, but also on their ideas as to what is or isn't harmful. It's also possible for young people to feel guilty about doing something that few people would consider harmful at all. For instance, one sixteen-year-old girl wrote to us:

> If I just kiss a boy goodnight I feel so ashamed, not while I'm kissing but afterwards. I know it's not normal to feel so guilty, yet I do. How can I get over feeling so guilty?
>
> *Frances, age 16*

This girl felt guilty and ashamed simply for kissing a boy goodnight. And, judging from the letters we get, she's not alone. Some kids feel guilty even though they haven't actually *done* anything at all. For example, some boys have told us that they felt not just shy or embarrassed, but also ashamed, of the fact that they've had wet dreams.

Kids may feel ashamed or guilty about their sexuality even though they haven't done anything harmful. If so, they may find it helpful to think about *why* they feel this way. Often it's because some important person (often a parent) or group (maybe a religion) has taught them to feel this way. At one time many people in our society had *very* negative attitudes about sexuality. In your great grandparents' day, sexual thoughts and feelings were often considered evil, the work of the devil. Sexual desires were considered impure or unclean, especially in women. Women who felt sexual urges or who enjoyed sex were considered abnormal, or perverted. Many people felt it was sinful even for married people to have sex, unless they were trying to have a child.

Of course, times change and so do people's attitudes. Today, most people in our society have more positive attitudes about sexuality. Still, many people continue to have negative, or at least somewhat negative, attitudes about sexuality. Parents who have these attitudes may pass them on to their children. Even though parents may not actually come out and say "sexuality is bad," they may pass these attitudes on in other ways. A parent might, for instance, get upset when a little baby touches his or her sex organs and move the baby's hands away or even slap them. This may give the baby the idea that sex organs are "nasty" or "dirty" and that it's "wrong" or "bad" to touch them. When that baby grows up, he or she may feel ashamed about menstruation or wet dreams or may feel guilty about masturbating.

When you think about it this way, it's really not surprising that some kids feel unnecessary guilt about their sexuality. They feel guilty even though they haven't actually done anything that is harmful to themselves or others. It can be very difficult for these young people to let go of their guilty feelings, but being aware of where these feelings come from can help. People can and do learn to work past their guilt.

SEXUAL CRIMES

When we talk about making sexual decisions in class, I often find questions about sexual crimes in the "Everything You Ever Wanted to Know" question box. You, too, may have questions about these things.

Parents sometimes don't talk with their children about sexual crimes because they don't want to scare them. Many parents want to protect their children from even hearing about such terrible things. This is understandable, but the fact of the matter is, sexual crimes do happen. We feel that it's better for children to know about sexual crimes. Then they can be prepared to handle a situation where they might be victims of a sexual crime.

Rape

Rape means forcing someone to have sex against his or her will. It can happen to anyone, to young children, to adults, to people of any age. Most rape victims are females, and most rapists are males. However, it's possible for a boy or man to be raped. Sometimes a male is raped by another male.

If you are a victim of rape, the most important thing is to get help right away. Some rape victims are so upset by what's happened that they just want to go home and try to forget the whole thing, but a rape victim needs medical attention as soon as possible. Even if the victim doesn't seem to have any serious injuries, there could be internal injuries that need medical attention. The victim also needs to be tested to make sure that he or she hasn't gotten a sexually transmitted disease. (These tests are one reason why a victim shouldn't bathe or shower before seeking medical attention.) If the victim is a female who is at least part of the way through puberty, she might want to take the morning-after pill to prevent pregnancy. (Girls have gotten pregnant even though they have not yet had their first periods.) A rape victim also needs support to recover emotionally as well as physically, and should seek help for this reason, too.

If you are a rape victim, there are a number of ways to go about getting help. You can go to a hospital emergency room or call 911 and the police will take you to the hospital. There are rape hotlines in most big towns and cities. You can find the number of the hotline closest to your home in your telephone directory or by calling the information operator.

Child Sexual Abuse

Child sexual abuse may involve anything from touching, feeling, fondling, or kissing the sex organs to actual sexual intercourse. Incest is one type of sexual abuse. It involves one member of a family being sexual with another family member. Of course, it isn't incest when a husband and wife do these things with each other. Also, brothers and sisters often engage in some form of sex play as they're growing up. This may involve "playing doctor" or pretending to be "mommy and daddy." This kind of sex play between young children is very common. It isn't usually considered incest and it isn't usually a harmful thing. But sexual contact between older siblings or with other family members is incest, and it can be very harmful.

Most victims of incest are girls who are victimized by their fathers, stepfathers, brothers, uncles, or some other male relatives. It is also possible for a girl to be victimized by a female relative. Boys can also be victims of incest. When incest happens to a boy, it may be either a female or a male relative who victimizes him. Incest can happen to very young children, even to babies, as well as to older children and teenagers.

Incest isn't always a forced thing, like rape. An older person in the family may be able to pressure the child into doing sexual things without actually having to use force. Most incest victims are so bewildered by what's going on that they simply don't know how to stop it or prevent it from happening again.

Child sexual abuse is considered incest only when the abuser is a family member. But sexual abuse can also occur when the abuser is a family friend, a teacher, a coach, a parent's boyfriend or girlfriend, another adult the victim knows, or even a complete stranger. Boys as well as girls may be victims of this type of sexual abuse.

If you are a victim of sexual abuse, the most important thing to do is to tell someone. This can be a difficult thing to do, particularly if you are an incest victim.

The logical people to tell are your parents. (Of course, in cases of incest by a parent, you need to tell the other parent.) However, some parents have trouble believing their children at first. If, for whatever reason, your parent won't believe you, you might tell another relative, an aunt or uncle, a grandparent, an older sister or brother, whom you feel will believe you. Or you could tell another adult, a teacher or counselor at school, a friend's mother or father, your minister or priest or rabbi, or any other adult you trust.

You can also call the Child Abuse Hotline. Their telephone number is listed in the Resource Section on page 231. The people who answer the phones there are specially trained and they understand what you're going through. (Some of them have been victims of sexual crimes themselves.) You don't have to give your name, and what you say is entirely confidential, so don't hesitate to call.

Victims of incest and other types of childhood sexual abuse often find it hard to come forward and tell someone. Sometimes the person who committed the crime has made the victim promise to keep it a secret, but there are some promises and some secrets a person needn't keep, and this is definitely one of them. The victims may also find it hard to tell someone because they think that what happened is somehow their fault. They think they're to blame because they didn't stop it from happening. This just isn't true. These crimes are always the fault of the older person. *The victim is never to blame and is never at fault in any way.* Some victims don't tell because they are afraid the person will harm them or get back at them for telling, but the police or other authorities will do whatever they can to protect the victim.

Incest victims sometimes hesitate to tell because telling could get the person who has committed the crime into trouble with the police. Even though most victims hate what's been done to them, some of them still don't want to see a relative sent to jail. Although involving the police may seem like a horrifying idea, it will be better for everyone in the end. It may protect any brothers or sisters who may also be suffering abuse. Besides, those who commit incest aren't always sent to jail. If possible the judge sends the person for some form of psychiatric treatment, while at the same time making sure that you are protected from further abuse.

Some incest victims don't tell because they're afraid that the family will break up. They fear that their parents will get divorced, or things will get worse than they are. But, if incest is going on, things are already about as bad as they could be. The victim and the other family members also need help in dealing with the situation. However, no one can get the help they need unless the victim has the courage to take the first step and tell someone.

Most victims of incest and other types of sexual abuse feel a mixture of anger, embarrassment, and shame. This can also make it hard to come forward and tell someone. But you have the right to protect yourself from abuse. So even though you may feel embarrassed, it's important to tell someone. It's really the best thing for everyone.

If you have been abused, you may have concerns about what will happen when you grow up and choose to begin having sex. Many victims worry that future sex partners will be able to tell that they've been abused. But this is not the case. No one will know about the abuse unless you choose to tell that person.

Being abused does not physically impair your sexual ability, but abuse can have long-lasting emotional effects. If you've been abused, we strongly suggest you get counseling to help you recover emotionally. (You can call the abuse hotline number listed in the Resource Section on page 231 for help in finding counseling in your area.)

A FEW FINAL WORDS

As you know, there are a number of physical changes that take place in our bodies during puberty. For most of us, these physical changes are accompanied by certain emotional changes. For instance, we may feel very "up," proud, and excited by the fact that we're growing up and becoming adults. But along with these positive feelings, most of us also experience less-than-totally-wonderful feelings from time to time as we're going through puberty. It's not uncommon for young people to have the "blues," times when we feel depressed or down in the dumps, sometimes for no apparent reason. Part of the reason we have these feelings may be the new hormones our bodies are making. Hormones are powerful substances, and they can affect our emotions. It takes our bodies and emotions some time to adjust to these hormones, and some doctors feel that the emotional ups and downs many people experience are due, at least in part, to hormonal changes. But it's undoubtedly more than that. It's not just our bodies that are changing, it's our whole lives. At times, all this changing can seem a bit overwhelming, and we may feel uncertain, scared, anxious, or depressed.

One girl wrote to my daughter and me after she'd read the girl's book on puberty, expressing feelings that a lot of kids share. She said:

> I'm going through puberty right now and I'm very scared about it. Everyone says it's normal to feel this way, but every time I'm feeling good and everything, I suddenly get this depressed feeling and I don't want to grow up anymore. I just never want to get older and face things like possible rapes, diseases, deaths, etc.
>
> Also, I'm going to my first year of junior high school and I'm really scared. I'm not sure I'm ready to face all the changes.

It is quite normal to have these kinds of feelings. Knowing that other kids your age have the same feelings won't magically make you feel better, but it can help you to know that at least you're not alone.

Sometimes, young people are upset because they feel pressured to grow up all at once. As one boy put it:

> Everyone I know is trying to grow up as fast as possible. What's the rush? I'm just not in a great big rush. I want to take my time. I'm tired of everyone trying to act all big and grown-up all the time.

And sometimes, the idea of being more grown-up and independent can be kind of scary. As one boy said:

> Okay, so now all of a sudden I'm supposed to be all grown-up and have all these adult responsibilities. But I'm not ready to have these responsibilities and make all these decisions. In a few years, I'm going to go to college or maybe get a job and live on my own, and I don't even know what I want to do or if I can really do everything on my own. Sometimes I just want to stay a little kid.

However, there may be times when we feel that people around us, especially our parents, are keeping us from growing up as fast as we'd like to. One teenage girl expressed this point of view:

> Sometimes I really hate my parents. They treat me like a little kid. They want to tell me what to wear or how I should wear my hair and where I can go and who I can go with and when I have to be home and blah, blah, blah. They're always bugging me. It's like they want me to stay "their little girl" forever and they won't let me grow up.

Going through puberty and becoming a teenager doesn't necessarily mean that you and your parents will have problems getting along with each other, but most teens do run into at least some conflicts with their parents. Indeed, at times it can seem like out-and-out war. These conflicts between teens and parents have to do with the change that takes place in the relationship between the parent and the child during these years. When we're little babies, we can't even feed ourselves, change our clothes, or go to the bathroom by ourselves. Our parents have to feed us, dress us, and change our diapers; we are *dependent* on them for everything. It's our parents' job to teach us how to take care of ourselves so that, eventually, we'll be able to go out and live on our own. And they have to take care of us and protect us until we're old enough to do that for ourselves. Children need their parents, but they also want to grow up, to be more independent, to take care of themselves, and to make decisions on their own. At the beginning of your teen years, you are still very dependent, but in a few years you'll be off to college or out earning your own living. So during your teen years, you and your parents are ending a relationship in which you're very dependent, and trying to establish a new relationship in which you are totally independent.

It's not easy to let go of old, familiar ways of relating and to establish new ones. Parents are used to being in charge, to making decisions. They may continue to tell you how to dress, how to wear your hair, what to do, and when to do it, even after you feel that you're old enough to make these decisions on your own. This change in the relationship from dependent to independent doesn't usually come off without a hitch. It can cause much of the stress, anger, and other negative feelings that you may experience during your teen years.

Our relationships with our friends also change during these years, and here again, this changing can cause uncertain, confused, depressed, or otherwise difficult emotional feelings. Chances are you'll begin junior high and be going to a new school, making new friends, perhaps seeing less of old friends. Breaking old ties and making new ones isn't always an easy thing to do. During these years, being part of a certain gang or group usually becomes a very important part of your life. It can make things easier and more fun. But groups can present problems, too. You may find that you aren't accepted into a certain "in" group even though you'd very much like to be a part of it. Feelings of being "out of it" or being excluded from the group can make things seem very lonely.

Even if you are accepted by the group, you may find that there are still some problems. Being part of a group can have a lot of rewards—it helps us feel more accepted, more a part of things, less lonely and uncertain. But sometimes being part of a group "costs" us. We may have to act in certain ways or do certain things we don't feel good about in order to stay part of the group. Here's what some kids had to say about this:

> I really want to be "in" with this group of kids at school, but they do some things I don't like. Like they're always laughing at kids who aren't in the group, making jokes or comments and stuff when one of those kids gets up in front of class or something. I really want to be accepted, and it's not like I have to do what they do to be accepted. But if I do, I don't feel good about myself.
>
> *Margie, age 14*

> I hate school 'cause I either have to act a certain way or be some outcast. Like in class, if you have an idea about something that is different than everyone else's, you can't say it or you'll be out of it and everyone will put you down. You have to do and say the same thing as everyone else or you're not okay.
>
> *Tim, age 13*

> Friends can talk me into doing things I don't really want to do. I'm in with the really "in" crowd, but the kids I run around

with drink and sometimes smoke dope 'cause that's cool. My parents would kill me if they knew what I do, and really I'm not so into these things, but I do them to be part of the group.

Sharon, age 15

Growing up is indeed a mixed bag of experiences. On the one hand, there are a lot of exciting things to look forward to; on the other hand, there are lots of changes—physical changes, life changes, changes in our relationships with our parents, our friends, and with the opposite sex. Probably at some time there must have been someone, somewhere, who went through puberty and the teenage years without a single problem, but we wouldn't bet a whole lot of money on it. If you're like most kids, you'll run into some problems as you go through the physical and emotional changes of puberty. We hope that this book will help in dealing with these problems. But this book is only a beginning; we've included a list of some other books we think you'll find helpful.

RESOURCE SECTION

In this section you'll find books, websites, hotlines, and organizations you can contact for help or further information about topics covered in this book. The resources are organized under the following headings:

- Birth Control, AIDS, and Other Sexually Transmitted Diseases (STDs)
- Circumcision
- Counseling and Therapy
- Eating Disorders: Anorexia, Bulimia, and Overeating
- Gay and Lesbian Youth
- Resources for Parents and Teachers
- Sexual Harassment and Abuse

A NOTE ABOUT THE INTERNET

The sources in this section include Internet websites and email addresses. All of us, and especially young people, need to be careful when we use the Internet. There are "adult only" websites with lewd and offensive material. If you find yourself at such a website, leave that website. Many websites are really businesses that are trying to part you from your money. So, *never give any business on the Internet a credit card number without first getting your parents' permission*. Also, don't fill out questionnaires that ask for personal information like your age, phone number, and address.

You can also talk directly to other people via Internet chatrooms and email. Many people find this an entertaining way to correspond with other people, but this can be dangerous. Remember anyone you talk to on the Internet is a complete stranger. They may not be anything like the person they say they are. Here are some common sense rules for staying out of trouble.

- Never give your last name, address, internet password, telephone number, or credit card number to someone you "talk to" on the Internet. Don't tell anyone what school you attend, where you go to church or temple, where you hang out, or any other information that could help someone find you. Immediately stop corresponding with anyone who asks for this kind of information.
- Never agree to meet someone you "talk to" on the Internet.
- Immediately stop corresponding with anyone who uses "nasty" language or in any other way makes you feel uncomfortable.
- If you're upset or puzzled by something that happens on the Internet, talk about it with a parent or some other adult that you trust.

The Internet is a marvelous source of information. So follow the rules and be safe.

Birth Control, AIDS, and Other Sexually Transmitted Diseases (STDs)

Changing Bodies, Changing Lives: A Book for Teens on Sex and Relationships by Ruth Bell and others (Random House, 1998).

This is a great book for older teens. There are excellent chapters on birth control and sexually transmitted diseases. (Be sure you get the 3rd edition, published in 1998 so you have the most up to date information.) The book also deals with a wide range of other issues, including sexuality, eating disorders, substance abuse, emotional health care, and safer sex.

Planned Parenthood (national office)
810 Seventh Avenue
New York, NY 10019
Phone: 212-541-7800
Website: http://www.plannedparenthood.org
Hotline Number: 800-230-7526

Planned Parenthood also has local chapters across the country. They provide birth control, pregnancy testing, testing and treatment for sexually transmitted diseases, abortion services or referrals, and other reproductive health information and services. You can call their 800 number for a clinic near you. Or look in the yellow pages under the headings family planning or birth control. Even if there's no Planned Parenthood clinic in your area, these headings should include listings for clinics that offer similar services to teens.

STD Hotlines
800-227-8922 (The National STD Hotline)
800-653-4325 (recorded STD information)
The National STD Hotline answers questions about any type of STD. You can also request pamphlets or other written information. In addition this hotline provides references for testing and treatment. The second number listed above provides recorded information about various STDs.

AIDS Hotlines
English: 800-342-2437
Spanish: 800-344-7432
Deaf Access: 800-243-7880
These hotlines will answer questions and you can also request written information.

Circumcision

The American Academy of Pediatrics (AAP)
141 Northwest Point Boulevard
Elk Grove Village, IL 60007
Phone: 847-228-5005
Fax: 847-228-5097
Website: http://www.aap.org/policy/re9850.html
        http://www.aap.org/family/circ.htm
AAP has a task force on circumcision. Their most recent policy statement is available online at the first website address above. They have information for parents at the second of the websites above.

The National Organization of Circumcision Information
Resource Centers
P.O. Box 2512
San Anselmo, CA 94979
Phone: 415-488-9883
Fax: 415-488-9660
Website: http://www.nocirc.org

You can get a referral to a doctor "educated about the function of the foreskin" and information about circumcision from this organization.

Doctors Opposing Circumcision (D.O.C.)
2442 NW Market Street, Suite 42
Seattle, Washington, 98107Phone: 813-657-9404
Email: gcd@u.washington.edu
Website: http://faculty.washington.edu/gcd/DOC
This organization is another good source for information about circumcision.

COUNSELING AND THERAPY

You don't have to deal with difficult emotional situations all by yourself. Difficult situations are a lot easier to deal with when you go outside yourself for help. There are many ways to find people who will listen to you and help you. You can talk to a parent or relative, to a friend, to a teacher, to a rabbi, minister, or priest.

There are also a number of ways to look for professional help in your area. Here are some:

- *Call a Hotline:* Look in the white pages under the headings: Teenline, Helpline, Talkline, Crisis Hotline, Crisis Intervention Services, and Suicide Prevention. If you can't find an appropriate hotline this way call a police station or a teen center and ask them for a hotline number. (You don't have to give then your name.) If you live in a small community with no hotlines then try the phone book of a large city in your area.
- *Contact a Teen Clinic:* Teen clinics often provide counseling services. Look in the yellow pages under Clinics. If you live in a small community with no teen clinics then try the phone book of a large city in your area.
- *Contact Your Church or Temple:* Ask your minister, priest, rabbi, or youth director to recommend a therapist or counselor.
- *Call a Radio Station:* Radio stations that broadcast mainly to teenagers or do talk-shows for teenagers, may be able to recommend a counseling service. You don't have to talk on the air, just call them and say you need help.
- *Ask Your Family Doctor:* Your family doctor should be able to recommend a therapist in your area.

- *Contact a Mental Health Center:* Mental Health Centers usually offer teen services. Look in the yellow pages under Clinic or Health Services. Also look in the white pages under your county services.
- *Call the American Psychological Association:* This organization will give you a referral to a psychologist in your area. Their referral number is: 1-800-924-2000.

EATING DISORDERS: ANOREXIA, BULIMIA, AND OVEREATING

American Anorexia Bulimia Association, Inc. (AABA)
165 West 46th Street, Suite 1108
New York, NY 10036
Phone: 212-575-6200
Website: http://www.aabainc.org
AABA provides information and referrals for support groups and treatment of anorexia, bulimia, and binge eating disorders. For referrals to resources in your area call the national office in New York during business hours (Eastern Standard Time). You can also request referrals via email. Include your state, zip code, and the name of the nearest major city.

National Association of Anorexia Nervosa and
Associated Disorders (ANAD)
P.O. Box 7
Highland Park, IL 60035
Hotline: 847-831-3438
Fax: 847-433-4632
Email: anad20@aol.com
Website: http://www.anad.org
ANAD is the oldest, national, nonprofit organization helping eating disorder victims and their families. It offers free counseling and information via hotline and email. (Their hotline number, however, is not a toll-free number.)

In addition, ANAD offers free referrals to therapists and treatment programs across the United States and operates a network of support groups for sufferers and families. The organization publishes a quarterly newsletter and will mail customized information packets upon request.

Overeaters Anonymous (OA)
P.O. Box 92870
Los Angeles, CA 90009
Email: sponsor@overeaters.org
Website: http://www.overeaters.org

OA is a self-help group based on the same twelve-step recovery program as Alcoholics Anonymous. There are no dues or fees to join or attend meetings. Their website contains information on OA and will help you find a meeting place near you. You can also email them with any questions you have. Or call the nearest OA chapter for information and local meeting times. (Look in the white pages under Overeaters Anonymous.)

Gay and Lesbian Youth

Campaign to End Homophobia
P.O. Box 819
Cambridge, MA 02139

This organization puts out two excellent pamphlets: "I Think I Might Be Gay . . . Now What Do I Do?" and "I Think I Might Be Lesbian . . . Now What Do I Do?" You can write to the above address for a single copy of either pamphlet. (Include a self-addressed, business-size envelope that is stamped for two ounces of postage. Contributions to the Campaign, to defray the costs of developing and distributing this material, are always welcomed.) These pamphlets are also available online at the website of the Youth Assistance Organization (YOA). (YOA is another excellent resource for gay and lesbian youth.) Their website address is http://www.youth.org.

GLB Teen Hotline: 800-347-TEEN

This hotline for gay, lesbian, and bisexual youth is available 7pm–10pm (Eastern Standard Time) Fridays and Saturdays.

Parents, Families, and Friends of Lesbians and Gays (PFLAG)
1101 14th Street, NW, Suite 1030
Washington, DC 20005
Phone: 202-638-4200
Website: http://www.pflag.org

PFLAG is a national support organization with chapters throughout the country. Some of their excellent pamphlets are available at their website. Their pamphlet "Be Yourself" can also be ordered by mail. Send $1.80 for each pamphlet and request a free information packet and list of publications.

Young, Gay and Proud by Don Romesburg (Alyson Publications, Fourth edition, 1995).

This is an excellent sourcebook for young people coming to terms with their sexuality.

RESOURCES FOR PARENTS AND TEACHERS

Many of the resources listed under other headings in this section will also be helpful for parents and teachers. Under this heading, I've listed a few of my favorite resources for parents and teachers.

ETR Associates
P.O. Box 1830
Santa Cruz, CA 95061
Phone: 800-321-4407
Website: http://www.etr.org

ETR publishes and distributes sexuality and health education materials for educators and parents, including books, curricula, brochures, videos, and other resources. I especially like "New Methods for Puberty Education—Grades 4–9" and their brochures and videos. You can browse their catalog online and write or call for a free catalog.

From Diapers to Dating: A Parent's Guide to Raising Sexually Healthy Children by Debra W. Haffner (Newmarket Press, 1999).

This book is filled with sound, sensible advice and guidelines that will enable parents to deal wisely with a whole gamut of sexuality issues.

Hostile Hallways: The AAUW Survey on Sexual
Harassment in America's Schools (AAUW, 1993).

This is the American Association of University Women's eye-opening survey on school sexual harassment.

How to Talk So Kids Will Listen and Listen So Kids Will Talk by Adele Faber and Elaine Mazlish (Avon Books, reissue edition, 1991).

Teaches basic communication skills that are invaluable for both parents and teachers.

The Kinsey Institute New Report on Sex by June Reinisch with Ruth Beasly (St. Martin's Press, 1994).

This comprehensive, basic reference contains information on a number of topics including puberty, anatomy and physiology, sexual health, and sexuality across the life cycle.

National Information Center for Children and Youth
with Disabilities (NICHCY)
P.O. Box 1492
Washington, DC 20013
Phone: 800-695-0285
Email: nichcy@aed.org
Website: http://www.nichcy.org

NICHCY is the national information and referral center that provides information on disabilities and disability-related issues for families and educators, including resources about teaching sexuality issues to children with disabilities. You can also get personal responses to specific questions via email or phone.

P.E.T.: Parent Effectiveness Training by Dr. Thomas Gordon (New American Library Trade, reissued edition, 1990).

This classic parenting guide teaches communication skills of value to parents and educators.

Sexuality Information and Education Council
of the United States (SIECUS)
130 W. 42nd Street, Suite 350
New York, NY 10036
Phone: 212-819-9770
Website: http://www.siecus.org

SIECUS is a national sex education advisory group. They have extensive materials for parents and teachers. Some of their excellent annotated bibliographies, fact sheets and helpful brochures for parents are available online. You can also write or call for a catalog of their publications.

Sexual Harassment and Abuse

National Child Abuse Hotline:
800-422-4453 (800-4-A-CHILD)
800-244-4453 (800-2-A-CHILD;
TTY for hearing impaired)

This 24-hour hotline is set up to help young people and parents with any kind of abuse—sexual, emotional, or physical. You can talk to a trained person, just stay on the line! You don't have to give your name. The hotline also provides information and referrals regarding child abuse issues.

Equal Rights Advocates
1663 Mission Street, Suite 550
San Francisco, CA 94103
Phone: 415-621-0672
Fax: 415-621-6744
Hotline: 1-800-839-4ERA
Website: http://www.equalrights.org/SexHar/School/sh-scho.htm

This organization's website provides excellent information for young people and parents about school sexual harassment. They also have a free advice and counseling hotline. You can leave a message twenty-four hours a day and someone will return your call.

INDEX

(Page references in italics refer to illustrations.)

abrasive soaps and scrubs, 112, 113
abuse, sexual, 213–16
  resources for information on, 231
acne, 97, 108–15, 173–74
  blackheads, 108, 110, 112
  causes of, 108–10, 112
  food and, 112
  pimples, 108, 110, *110,* 112,
    173–74
  treatment of, 111–15
  whiteheads, 108, 109, 110, 112
African-Americans, skin concerns
  for, 113
AIDS, 207
  resources for information on,
    224–25
alcohol, 93
aluminum, 107
anorexia, resources for information
  on, 227–28
antiperspirants, 107–8
anus, *6,* 8, 12, 152
appearance, fashions in, 94–96, *95*
areola, 117, *117*
arousal, 152
athletic supporters, 144, 145, *145*

babies, making, 5, 13, 15–21, *21,*
  127, 177
bathing, 68, 106
benzoyl peroxide, 111–12
birth control, 204–5
  resources for information on,
    224–25
bisexuality, 194
blackheads, 108, 110, 112

bladder, *129,* 133, 135, 136
blue, feeling, 217
body odor, 97–98, 105–8
body proportions, changes in:
  in boys, 3, 82–84, *83*
  in girls, 173
body types, 85–86, *85*
bones, 74, 80, 88, 89, 92, 93
bowel movements, 8
bras, 168–69
breasts:
  female, 167–69, *168, 170,* 172
  male, 117–19
buffered aluminum sulfate, 107
bulimia, resources for information
  on, 227–28

calcium, 89–92, 93
cancer, 70, 119, 140–43
cervix, 134, *177*
child sexual abuse, 213–16
  resources for information on, 231
circumcision, 9, *10,* 54, *55,* 56–57,
  61, 64–66
  resources for information on,
    225–26
  scars from, 64–66, *66*
clitoris, *6,* 12, 52, 174
  slang words for, 13
clothing, perspiration and, 106, 107
condoms, 205
corona, 54, *55,* 63, 64, 67, 68
counseling, resources for, 226–27
Cowper's glands, 128, *129,* 130, 135,
  138
cramps, menstrual, 184

Lynda Madaras Books for Pre-Teens and Teens (and Their Families, Friends, and Teachers)

Order from your local bookstore or write or call:
Newmarket Press, 18 East 48th Street, New York, NY 10017;
(212) 832-3575 or (800) 669-3903; Fax (212) 832-3629;
E-mail sales@newmarketpress.com

Please send me the following books by Lynda Madaras:

THE WHAT'S HAPPENING TO MY BODY? BOOK FOR GIRLS
_____ copies at $22.95 each (gift hardcover)
_____ copies at $12.95 each (trade paperback)

THE WHAT'S HAPPENING TO MY BODY? BOOK FOR BOYS
_____ copies at $22.95 each (gift hardcover)
_____ copies at $11.95 each (trade paperback)

MY BODY, MY SELF FOR GIRLS
_____ copies at $12.95 each (trade paperback)

MY BODY, MY SELF FOR BOYS
_____ copies at $12.95 each (trade paperback)

MY FEELINGS, MY SELF (A Growing-Up Guide For Girls}
_____ copies at $12.95 each (trade paperback)

For postage and handling, add $3.00 for the first book, plus $1.00 for each additional book. Please allow 4-6 weeks for delivery. Prices and availability subject to change.

I enclose a check or money order, payable to Newmarket Press, in the amount of $_____.(NY residents please add sales tax.)

Name _____

Address _____

City/State/Zip _____

Special discounts are available for orders of five or more copies. For information, contact Newmarket Press, Special Sales Dept., 18 East 48th Street, New York, NY 10017;
(212) 832-3575 or (800) 669-3903; Fax (212) 832-3629 ;
E-mail sales@newmarketpress.com